Anti-Inflammatory Guide and Cookbook for Beginners

Heal Your Immune System and Balance Your Body

Table of Contents

Introduction

The health of a human being is intrinsically linked to the health of their internal organs. These organs are constantly in contact with the external environment, which is largely polluted and infested with bacteria, viruses, parasites, and other pathogens. Any microorganism that comes into contact with a human being has a chance of entering its body and making them sick.

The human immune system prevents infection by defending the body against foreign invaders; this process contributes to our overall health. Therefore, if a person is not healthy, it can be assumed that their immune system is not working properly.The inflammatory response is the first line of defense against foreign invaders and plays an important role in wound healing. However, inflammation occurs when tissue is damaged and contributes to the pain response when a person suffers from injury or illness.

The inflammatory response can be a good thing if it helps the body heal quickly and if it does not harm healthy tissue as it works to repair the damage, but there are cases where inflammation does more harm than good. Chronic inflammation can develop if the immune system becomes excessively sensitive and begins attacking itself. Since the inflammatory response is responsible for immune system regulation, this can lead to various health issues down the road. Chronic inflammation also increases the risk of cardiovascular disease and every kind of cancer.

Chronic inflammation does not occur overnight; it develops over time due to poor lifestyle habits and repeated exposure to environmental toxins. The foods we eat, the air we breathe, and our drinking water can all cause chronic inflammation. Being overweight or obese is another risk factor because fat tissue releases inflammatory chemicals like cytokines into the body. An imbalanced microbiome can also contribute towards chronic inflammation because healthy gut flora help regulates immune responses by producing anti-inflammatory compounds called "competence factors.

While chronic inflammation is not a condition that can be cured, it can be managed by making lifestyle changes. Eating an anti-inflammatory diet, incorporating stress-reducing activities, and removing toxins from the home and body are all essential steps toward getting to the root cause of chronic inflammation. This guide will help you understand the basics of chronic inflammation and how you can manage it; it provides information on anti-inflammatory foods, supplements, and lifestyle habits that you can use to your advantage in your journey toward overall health.

Numerous chronic disorders, including leukemia, lymphoma, Alzheimer's disease, and rheumatoid arthritis, are all made more likely by chronic inflammation. The cause of chronic inflammation is largely unknown, but it is a complex condition that can be traced back to a combination of genetic predisposition and environmental factors.

It has been suggested that chronic inflammation may be the result of two separate yet interconnected processes: one is the ability of our immune system to carry out an anti-inflammatory response, and the other process is a "self-perpetuating" process that leads to overreaction by an already hyperactive immune response. In the case of an imbalance in the immune response, there is an overproduction of pro-inflammatory cytokines, which can cause damage to normal tissue and contribute to chronic inflammation.

The interplay between these two processes is unclear; however, research suggests that genetic predisposition (specifically genes involved in immune response regulation) may be a key factor. It has been documented that families with a history of inflammatory conditions are more likely to develop them than those without a family history.

In conditions like rheumatoid arthritis and multiple sclerosis, it has been found that those who have a genetic predisposition are more likely to develop an inflammatory condition whether or not they have the disease. The presence of chronic inflammation does not always mean there is a genetic predisposition towards it; however, research has shown that high rates of inflammation do occur in families with a history of autoimmune diseases.

Inflammation is identified by irritation on specific parts of the body. This irritation can happen through injury or from an overreaction by our immune system; it can also come from environmental hazards such as pollutants or harmful bacteria. When an area of the body becomes irritated, white blood cells go to the area in an attempt to fight off any harmful substances. This triggers inflammation because more white blood cells are accumulating than are needed at that specific site.

In addition to genetics and environmental factors, other proposed contributors include infection, stress/anxiety, heart disease risk medications, and alcohol metabolism. Certain infections, such as tuberculosis and hepatitis C may trigger chronic inflammation in those who are already predisposed or who were previously exposed to these viruses.

Stress and anxiety can also cause chronic inflammation, though the extent to which it causes chronic inflammation is unclear. Studies have shown that those who suffer from more psychological stress are more likely to develop a condition such as inflammatory bowel disease (IBD) than those who lead relatively peaceful lives.
In addition, studies have shown that people with IBD tend to be anxious and depressed, which makes them more susceptible to developing chronic inflammation in the body.

Chronic inflammation is also linked with heart disease risk factors. The link between chronic inflammation and an individual's exposure to developing heart disease depends on the particular risk factor in question.

For example, cigarettes or smoking, in general, increases the possibility of chronic inflammation, which can increase the risk of developing heart disease. Research shows that smokers have a higher level of circulating inflammatory cytokines than non-smokers, and it also shows that smoking cessation leads to lower levels of inflammation.

Medications used for diabetes (i.e., metformin) and hypertension increase the likelihood of an imbalance in the immune response, which can lead to chronic inflammation. Studies show that these medications, in addition to stress, can increase levels of cytokines in the body. Alcohol metabolism also contributes to chronic inflammation; however, the exact relationship between alcohol and chronic inflammation is unclear.

On the one hand, research shows that excessive alcohol intake leads to high levels of circulating cytokines. However, it is also possible that those who are prone to inflammatory conditions are simply more likely to drink alcohol excessively or become addicted to it.

Studies have found that levels of acute phase reactants (e.g., CRP) rise with age and tend to be elevated among those who suffer from chronic conditions such as cardiovascular disease or diabetes mellitus type 2.

This book will take you deep into the world of inflammation and how to control it. It will teach you to control your diet by following specific rules to help keep chronic inflammation in control.

It will also teach you about supplements that can help reduce inflammation and support your immune system. It is time for you to take a stance against chronic inflammation by following the tips laid out in this book. Remember, prevention is key, and the first step to eliminate chronic inflammation starts with you.

Chapter 1: What Is Inflammation?

It is a natural response of the body to injury or infection. The body responds to inflammation by sending a wide variety of chemicals, known as biochemical mediators, into the area where it is injured or infected. These mediators help fight off any infection, remove dead tissue, and repair damaged tissue.

Although inflammation was originally believed to be an undesirable side effect of healing injuries, substantial data indicate that this process is necessary for normal wound healing and proper recovery from surgery. It is believed that excess inflammation will have a negative effect on several physiological processes in the body during exercise.

There also have been several studies that indicate that levels of inflammation can be enhanced by a number of prescriptions and over-the-counter medications taken by many athletes. Inflammation is sometimes used to refer to the process of all cellular events associated with an immune response, such as the production of white blood cells, the formation of antibodies, and the activation of macrophages.

Common symptoms of inflammation

The common pain and fever signs of inflammation are;

1. Heat: When inflammation starts, the body releases chemicals that cause heat. This is to prevent infection and kill bacteria or other organisms causing infection. The heat produced is usually described as a burning sensation.

2. Redness: The body also produces a chemical that causes the area to become visible by the red coloring. The red color appears because these extra blood cells are darker than normal (hence the purple color), and they also have more hemoglobin, which is why they appear reddish-brown.

Blood flow to the area becomes more rapid but less efficient (hence these capillaries are sometimes filled with extra fluid), so there is increased leakage of fluid into tissues.

3. Swelling: Blood vessels open wider than usual and allow more blood to come into the affected area. This allows white blood cells and other substances in the blood to come into contact with bacterial or foreign organisms at the site of injury or infection if any exist.

Unexplained swelling can be caused by any number of inflammatory conditions, such as rheumatism, deep bruising, and edema associated with heart failure or a kidney disorder.

4. Pain: This is caused by chemicals that inflame tissues and cause a painful sensation. For example, the chemical bradykinin causes pain, itching, and inflammation by stimulating the production of prostaglandins, leukotrienes, histamine, and cytokines.

These chemicals also help the blood cells (white) to penetrate areas of infection and fight the infection. It can also make people avoid doing things that may cause pain in the future (e.g., drinking alcohol).

5. Loss of function: This is caused by the swelling of tissues, which can press on nerves or blood vessels and can squeeze out or prevent the flow of blood. Loss of function can be mild (not being able to bend a joint as far as one normally can) or severe (being partially or totally paralyzed).

Taking the mystery out of inflammation

An injury can cause an inflammatory response, but that doesn't always mean that the injury was a result of inflammation. This seems counter-intuitive, and it took researchers years to figure it out. For a long time, they thought that inflammation was the root of chronic problems with injuries. Now we know better since our understanding of arachidonic acid (AA) metabolism has helped us see the truth. Chronic inflammation is dangerous, and it is important to know the difference.

Inflammation, if uncontrolled, may lead to heart disease, diabetes, arthritis, or cancer. So why do people think they have high levels of inflammation? People can increase their production of chronic inflammation by taking over-the-counter medications (the ones that you read about in the media), eating a lot of processed foods, and being exposed to certain pollutants (such as air pollution).

The key to understanding inflammation is understanding its effects on arachidonic acid metabolism. This seemingly simple explanation outlines how most diseases are linked to inflammatory processes. Arachidonic Acid (ARA) is a cell signaling molecule found in the membranes of cells.

It serves many functions, but the most important is to protect the cell by preventing enzymes and other important molecules from being destroyed. However, when inflammation occurs, it is usually because of an injury. White blood cells need to be activated to help heal the damage caused by an injury or infection and prevent further damage (called an inflammatory response).

So how does inflammation cause pain and fever? Inflammation causes pain by activating nerve endings in muscles and joints that send pain signals to our brains. This becomes particularly dangerous if you injure yourself while playing or training. This often happens when you decelerate suddenly, such as in a powerful tackle or hit.

Once white blood cells (macrophages) detect an injury and get activated, they release enzymes that break down ARA. When these enzymes begin to break down ARA, they destroy specific proteins that are critical to muscle function, such as myosin and actin. This causes muscle weakness by decreasing the amount of tonus (strength) and causing pain in the muscles.

The association between inflammation and soreness was recently shown using MRI (magnetic resonance imaging). Researchers used functional MRI (fMRI) to find out how much white blood cells were being activated during different exercises.

The results showed that more inflammation occurred in the body after strenuous exercise. This means that people who train longer or harder have a greater inflammatory response.

Strenuous exercise makes your body dehydrated. This can explain why people become tired or notice muscle soreness after a hard workout. The dehydration also stimulates a stress response which causes heat and redness in the area.

Heat causes pain as well, so it is critical to avoid dehydration after strenuous exercise by drinking plenty of water or sports drinks with electrolytes like sodium and potassium (salt).

Difference between acute and chronic inflammation

Acute inflammation is caused by an acute injury. It produces symptoms for up to seven days and can be repaired. Chronic inflammation is caused by an ongoing injury or infection that has gone on for at least three weeks. In this condition, no symptoms disappear, and the problem persists – it is called 'chronic' because it never goes away completely.

Chronic inflammation contributes to many diseases and conditions, including diabetes. Chronic inflammation can be caused by a single, big acute injury (e.g., hitting your thumb with a hammer), by many small injuries that cause only minor pain (e.g., repeated small injuries in the form of sports or exercise injuries), or by diseases which damage cells and tissues and which the body continually tries to repair but is unable to.

Guidelines for an anti-inflammatory diet

Anti-inflammation refers to the process whereby the body uses high doses of antioxidants and antioxidants are typically found in foods like vegetables and fruits. Anti-inflammation is the opposite of auto-inflammatory, which causes damage to cells, tissues, and organs and ultimately can lead to chronic inflammatory conditions such as heart disease, diabetes, or arthritis.

A critical aspect of this natural healing process is preventing external factors that might cause inflammation due to pollution exposure or other environmental factors.

For diet, the nutritional regimen is critical. The more energy we expend during exercise, the more nutrients we need from our foods to replace lost electrolytes (sodium, potassium, and minerals). Hydration is also essential for muscle recovery.

What is an anti-inflammatory diet?

The anti-inflammatory diet is a specific kind of nutritional plan. It is a diet that contains foods beneficial for those affected by chronic inflammation. Foods included in this diet should have a high concentration of antioxidants, and phytonutrients. A diet that helps to control inflammation reduces the risk of chronic disease and promotes optimal health.

Anti-inflammatory foods

There are several foods you can introduce in your diet. These are:

1. Beans: Instant and dried black beans are excellent sources of protein and fiber. They also provide ample amounts of zinc and copper, plus other minerals such as manganese, phosphorus, and magnesium.

2. Chili Peppers: Red chili peppers are more anti-inflammatory than green ones, so opt for red peppers. Chilis are excellent holders of vitamin C and capsaicin, both powerful antioxidants and anti-inflammatory agents. Capsaicin has some interesting side effects, including reduced heart disease and cancer risk.

3. Turmeric: This South Asian spice is a powerhouse of anti-inflammatory nutrients, including curcumin. Studies have shown that taking capsules of curcumin can help reduce inflammation and support the healing process following a heart attack.

4. Oily fish: Wild salmon, tuna, and fresh sardines are some of the most effective ways of obtaining omega-3 fatty acids. These fatty acids can help to fight daily inflammation. The benefits include decreased risk of inflammatory diseases.

DHA, commonly known as (docosahexaenoic acid) is the major omega-3 fatty acid. It lowers blood pressure, acts as an anti-inflammatory agent, and positively affects blood sugar control in diabetics.

5. Nuts: Nuts such as walnuts, pine nuts, and almonds are high in anti-inflammatory antioxidants. They have been shown to help prevent heart disease and cancer inflammation.

6. Berries: Blueberries, blackberries, and strawberries are rich sources of anthocyanin antioxidants. These berries have been shown to have powerful anti-inflammatory effects that help prevent cancer, infection, heart disease, and stroke.

7. Seeds: Flaxseeds also contain omega-3 fatty acids. These seeds support heart health by lowering levels of triglycerides in the blood as well as helping to lower inflammation from chronic disease.

8. Seafood: Salmon, trout, sardines, and tuna are rich sources of omega-3s as well as vitamin D. These nutrients help to reduce inflammation.

9. Citrus: Oranges, lemons, grapefruits, and pomelo are rich sources of vitamin C. This powerful antioxidant helps to fight off inflammation by inhibiting the production of two pro-inflammatory enzymes in white blood cells called collagenase and MMP-9.

10. Avocados: These amazing fruits are an excellent source of monounsaturated fat (10g per avocado). They also have a high content of potassium, something that is critical for healthy blood pressure and fluid balance and for reducing blood cholesterol levels.

11. Dark chocolate: Dark chocolate is a rich source of flavonoids, and cacao contains powerful antioxidant substances called phenols. Studies have shown that when consumed, these antioxidants can assist in reducing inflammation, support heart health as well as helping to fight off chronic disease.

12. Garlic: This pungent ingredient can help to lower hypertension and minimize the possibility of many cardiac diseases by combating inflammation in the body. Also, garlic is a great source of anti-inflammatory sulfur compounds, including allicin, which is responsible for the smell and taste of garlic.

13. Herbs: Parsley, oregano, rosemary, and thyme are excellent sources, rich in nutrients of anti-inflammatory nature, including zinc, beta carotene, and vitamin C. Studies have shown that consuming these herbs can help fight off infections.

14. Oregano oil: This highly potent oil has been proven to have powerful anti-inflammatory properties and even has some antibiotic effects. It is believed that the main ingredient responsible for these effects is carvacrol which has been shown to significantly reduce symptoms of asthma in patients who consumed it for 30 days.

15. Green tea: Epigallocatechin-3-gallate aka (EGCG) is a powerful antioxidant contained in this tea; this powerful substance can help to prevent plaque buildup in the arteries.

16. Pomegranates: This fruit is a great source of the antioxidant hydroxytyrosol. Studies have shown that this antioxidant has powerful anti-inflammatory effects.

17. Cayenne: An ingredient found in chili peppers, this spice also has powerful anti-inflammatory properties. These properties include suppressing the production of pro-inflammatory prostaglandins and oxygen-free radicals.

18. Grapefruit: A sweet tropical fruit, grapefruit is a rich source of naringenin and hesperidin. These two antioxidants are powerful anti-inflammatory agents as they help to minimize body inflammation by counteracting the effects of two enzymes known as cyclooxygenase-2 (COX-2) and lipoxygenase (LO).

19. Ginger: This pungent ingredient has been shown to be an effective supplement for treating inflammatory conditions such as arthritis, lupus, and asthma. It is also effective at combating arterial inflammation, which can lead to heart disease and atherosclerosis.

20. Fennel: Fennel is an excellent source of anethole, a potent anti-inflammatory antioxidant. Studies have shown that fennel may help to treat inflammation in the respiratory tract, fight off allergies and boost immunity.

21. Skullcap: This herb is considered an effective treatment for several inflammatory conditions and is thought to work through the inhibition of COX-2 enzymes.

22. Paprika: This spice is a rich source of capsaicin which has been shown to have powerful properties (anti-inflammatory) for the skin and joints.

23. Fruits and vegetables - Rich in antioxidants and phytonutrients, fruits and vegetables are excellent sources of anti-inflammatory compounds. Some examples include berries, leafy greens, sweet potatoes, and broccoli.

24. Olive oil - Rich in monounsaturated fats and antioxidants, olive oil has been shown to have anti-inflammatory properties.

25. Leafy greens - Leafy greens such as kale, spinach, and collard greens are rich in vitamins and minerals that can help reduce inflammation.

26.Tart cherry juice - Contains antioxidants and anthocyanins that have been shown to have anti-inflammatory effects.

A healthy diet is optimal for a healthy body but doesn't forget that inflammation can be triggered by environmental factors like pollution or other external causes. A clean environment is imperative for healing the body and keeping it strong, so find ways to avoid pollution sources.

Also, eat plenty of fruits and vegetables that contain anti-inflammatory ingredients like broccoli, apples, and tomatoes, always wash them clean to get rid of any pesticide traces of the fruit or vegetable itself.

Anti-inflammatory diets are typically high in colorful fruits and vegetables, including blueberries, tomatoes, and watermelons. Other choices include bell peppers, leafy greens like spinach, kale, or collards, as well as cruciferous vegetables such as broccoli and Brussels sprouts.

It's important to note that some fruits contain a lot of sugar, so it's important to select those with less sugar, such as blueberries. The intake of whole fruits and vegetables can help reduce inflammation and the risk of chronic diseases.

On the protein side of things, focus on fish, chicken, and beans. These proteins are rich in anti-inflammatory flavonoids, including highly anti-inflammatory omega-3 fatty acids. Other choices include eggs, nuts, and seeds.

It is generally recommended to limit red meat and cut down on dairy in the diet. As for spices and herbs, ginger, turmeric, rosemary, cilantro, and thyme contain antioxidant properties that support anti-inflammatory diets.

Other foods to consider in your daily diet include fish oil supplements (DHA primarily), flaxseed oil, chia seeds, black currants, and borage seed oil. The best way to consume omega 3's is through their natural sources, which are usually fish or seafood, especially salmon and tuna.

Omega 3's are stored in the heart and brain, so in the case of chronic inflammation, focusing on those with a high source of omega-3 can help to reduce inflammation. Recent research suggests omega-3 can reduce the risk of cognitive decline and dementia due to its anti-inflammatory properties.

Another important addition to an anti-inflammatory diet is magnesium. Magnesium is a known anti-inflammatory and antioxidant, which can help reduce inflammation in the body. It is one of the most fundamental minerals in our diet since it affects nearly all cell functions.

Magnesium can be found in nuts, seeds, leafy greens, beans, and whole grains. Although it may seem tricky to reduce inflammation in the body, implementing anti-inflammatory changes into your daily diet is easy.

The main thing is to prevent inflammation from occurring, and adding anti-inflammatory foods to your diet can help aid that. Fruits and vegetables are the most important components of an anti-inflammatory diet.

Beyond that, there are ways to make simple changes that can help with inflammation. With the right amount of nutrients and a diet rich in anti-inflammatory foods, there is a very good chance you can prevent chronic diseases.

Studies on the impacts of diet in health and disease

A 2016 review of studies found that incorporating high animal fat, saturated fat, and cholesterol in your diet is linked with the growth of risk factors for cardiovascular diseases. It also found that a diet high in carbohydrates, including refined grains and added sugar, was associated not only with inflammatory diseases but also cancer.

Diet affects the core body temperature, and inflammation is linked to increased body temperature. Compounds in red meat, such as saturated fats, lower the body's core temperature by causing an increase in the heat generated by fat white cells. The metabolic changes triggered by inflammation can cause an increase in body temperature and an obvious association with higher temperatures and higher exposure to cancer.

Furthermore, there is convincing evidence that inflammation has a role in chronic disease, aging, and poor health outcomes. The liver produces C-reactive protein (CRP), which is utilized as a measure of chronic inflammation in response to tissue damage.

The main findings of the studies reviewed suggested that higher amounts of specific nutrients—like magnesium, vitamin D, omega-3 fatty acids, and phosphorus—were associated with lower levels of C-reactive protein in the blood.

Sugar intake is associated with increased blood levels of CRP. A 2016 review suggests that a high-sugar diet may increase systemic inflammation and the accumulation of visceral fat (between the organs) and increase the number or size of fatty liver lesions. Many studies have also suggested that consuming refined grains and sugar is rumored to increase the risk of C-reactive protein and lower magnesium readings.

A study published in 2011 suggested that consuming fructose at high doses can increase plasma levels of CRP. In addition, a diet high in sugar and refined carbohydrates has also been found to increase the risk of chronic diseases, including cardiovascular disease, cancer, diabetes, and obesity.

The body produces CRP from excess blood sugar produced by an overabundance of energy, eventually leading to cellular damage and inflammation. High-sugar diets are associated with increased C-reactive protein, but it is unclear whether the increased C-reactive protein is a mere marker of inflammation or if it contributes to the production of inflammatory markers.

All these studies point out that we need different types of foods to maintain our health and well-being; they need to be loaded with different nutrients such as antioxidants, fatty acids, and essential vitamins to protect against chronic diseases. In other words, we need a diet that is rich in anti-inflammatory foods.

Myths and facts

Here are the common myths about inflammation and reasons why you should not believe in these myths:

1. All inflammation is bad: This is not true. We have beneficial inflammation, and it has to do with healing tissues and creating new ones. It is not a disease but rather a normal process of the body. When the body is healthy, it produces certain proteins that help fight off infections and foreign substances.

When the body is unhealthy, this part of immunity turns into chronic inflammation that can damage tissues or organs. One example would be arthritis or carpal tunnel syndrome caused by an injury or illness to the joints or nerves. These are not normally harmful conditions, and they result in inflammatory responses that can heal the tissues and move the body toward health.

2. Gluten is inflammatory to everyone: We are different people, and everyone has different reactions to parts of our diet. Some people have more problems with dairy, wheat, soy, and other foods than others. Some people get a reaction after eating excessive portions of food that gives them "a headache" or other side effects.

Some people have no problems with gluten, but others react strongly to it (called celiac disease). It is a protein that gives dough its elasticity and structure. This process is called gluten forming, where the proteins found in foods such as gluten are rearranged when you cook or bake food. Research has shown that IBD can be triggered by foods high in protein, such as gluten and casein.

3. Eating nightshade vegetables will increase inflammation: People who believe this myth believe that all nightshade vegetables are bad for them. However, that's not the case. They contain anti-inflammatory compounds called flavonoids, which is why people with IBS want to avoid foods that are high in them, such as eggplant, peppers, potatoes, and tomatoes, since they tend to be anti-inflammatory.

However, some people have an excessive intake of these foods, which can be unhealthy. However, these foods can be eaten in small amounts without any negative effects on your body.

4. Eating low-carb offers more anti-inflammatory benefits: This is not the case since the body needs carbohydrates to produce energy. A person's metabolism can vary with their diet. Processed foods are higher in calories than whole foods, and low-carb diets may lead to weight gain because they are tough to stick to for the long term, and the person might rebound and eat excessive calories, which will result in more weight gain; usually, high-fat or high-protein diets lack many healthy carbohydrates such as vegetables, fruits, grains, beans, and seeds that help maintain energy levels, balance blood sugar and avoid overeating.

5. All sweet foods cause inflammation and spike blood sugar: This is false. This is a myth that started in the 60s and 70s when it was believed that all sugar is bad. Sugar can be found in many foods, and it doesn't change the amount of inflammation that you have.

However, studies have shown that foods with added sugars can spike your blood sugar, causing insulin resistance or diabetes. If a person has diabetes or insulin resistance, they are more likely to develop inflammation-related diseases such as heart disease and type 2 diabetes.

6. Plant-based omega-3 foods have the most anti-inflammatory benefits: Omega-3 foods can also be found in fish and plants. Salmon and other fish fats are considered anti-inflammatory, but plant-based omega-3 foods include pumpkin seeds, walnuts, flaxseed oils, soybeans, and canola oil. These oils help reduce inflammation by lowering markers associated with inflammation, such as C-reactive protein.

7. Following an anti-inflammatory diet means cutting a lot of foods out: When you follow an anti-inflammatory diet, you have so much freedom in what you can eat. Unlike other diets that restrict your foods, on an anti-inflammatory diet, you are not cutting out any food or food group. You are just restricting the number of foods that you intake.

8. Soy causes inflammation and should be avoided: Soy products are low in carbohydrates and caloric content, making them a good food to be included in your diet. However, the high estrogen content in soy may lead to hormonal imbalances that increase inflammation in some people. It is best to find out if you react to soy before eating it on a regular basis. If you do react to soy, it's best not to eat more than one serving per week or have other high-estrogen foods per week.

Chapter 2: Inflammation's Role in Chronic Disease

Chronic diseases are the most common and leading cause of death across all age groups. Chronic diseases are long-lasting, disabling, prevalent, and life-altering conditions that are characterized by a progressive impairment of organ functioning or structure.

Chronic diseases can be majorly categorized into two, autoimmune disorders and non-autoimmune inflammatory disorders (disorders not primarily associated with the immune system). There is a significant overlap between the two categories meaning both can be associated with chronic inflammation.

It is important to understand that there are various pathways involved in the development of inflammation, including genetic predisposition, environmental triggers, and diet. This presentation of pathophysiologic events may differ from individual to individual.

It is important to remember that inflammation is associated with many chronic diseases. As more research continues to be conducted into chronic diseases and inflammation, more evidence emerges that supports the association between chronic disease and inflammatory processes.

Chronic disease is not an isolated event but rather a chain of events leading to death and disability. This chain of events hinges upon numerous factors, including genetic predisposition, environmental triggers, and nutrition. Various pathways are involved in developing chronic inflammatory conditions. Genetic predisposition may be a significant contributor to the development of chronic disease because it can affect both environmental triggers and diet.

Genetic and environmental factors are believed to be involved in the pathophysiology of chronic disease. The process of chronic disease involves multiple factors and interactions between these factors, genetics, and the environment. It is important to understand that inflammation can significantly contribute to the development of chronic diseases.

Rheumatoid arthritis

This is a common inflammatory disorder and is characterized by joint inflammation. Research suggests that dietary influences can play a role in the progression of rheumatoid arthritis. There are food-related triggers that may increase the risk of developing rheumatoid arthritis; however, these triggers do not specifically cause the condition.

It appears that nutrition indirectly influences inflammatory processes rather than triggering them directly. In addition, environmental triggers can have an indirect influence on inflammation through diet. These triggers include smoking, infections, and certain foods or beverages to which individuals have a genetic predisposition.

Symptoms

The following are the symptoms and characteristic findings of rheumatoid arthritis:

• Joint pain: This is usually located around the joints of the body (wrists, fingers, shoulders, elbows, toes, and knees). The pain can range from intermittent to chronic. Individuals suffering from rheumatoid arthritis may also experience joint stiffness.

It is important to recognize that pain is a subjective experience; therefore, individuals can feel it differently. It has been reported that the possibility of developing rheumatoid arthritis is greater for individuals with a history of joint injury due to trauma or repetitive strain.

• Fever: Individuals can experience fever in association with the joint pain of rheumatoid arthritis. Individuals may also experience a fever that is not related to inflammation or joint pain.

• Weight loss: Individuals may experience weight loss associated with rheumatoid arthritis; however, excessive weight loss is not common. Weight loss relates primarily to the development of anemia.

• Fatigue: The combination of joint pain and fatigue makes it difficult for individuals to complete daily activities. This can lead to depression and the development of low self-esteem pertaining to daily tasks such as personal hygiene, washing dishes, or completing home chores.

• Weakness: As the joints of the body are inflamed, movement becomes limited. Individuals may also experience a tingling sensation or loss of function within the muscles of their hands and feet.

• Stiffness in the joint: Individuals experiencing rheumatoid arthritis may experience stiffness within the joint of the affected body part. The stiffness can be moderate or severe.

Treatment

There are multiple medical treatments that are used to manage joint pain associated with rheumatoid arthritis. The primary focus of these treatments is to minimize signs, improve function and restore mobility.

• Nonsteroidal anti-inflammatory medications: This type of medication is used to relieve inflammation and reduce pain associated with rheumatoid arthritis. Medications are typically prescribed for individuals who experience joint pain and stiffness that does not resolve or improve within 24 hours following activity or position changes.

In addition, nonsteroidal anti-inflammatory medications are often prescribed for individuals who experience continuous inflammation. These medications play a role in the treatment of rheumatoid arthritis; however, they do not cure the condition.

• Steroids: Individuals suffering from severe pain associated with rheumatoid arthritis may be prescribed steroids. This type of medication is for individuals who do not respond to the treatment of other drugs.

• Disease-modifying antirheumatic drugs (DMARDs): it is a form of medication helpful in slowing the advancement of rheumatoid arthritis, reducing the symptoms, and avoiding joint damage. The goal is to treat the symptoms associated with rheumatoid arthritis, improve mobility and maintain function.

When compared to others (NSAID), DMARDs drugs have been demonstrated to decrease joint damage and reduce inflammation. Disease-modifying antirheumatic drugs are primarily targeted toward specific symptoms or signs of rheumatoid arthritis, including pain, stiffness, or swelling in joints.

Asthma

Asthma is a long-term (chronic) condition in which the airways in the lungs become narrow and inflamed. The inflammation of the airways is characterized by bronchial hyperreactivity and spasms, mucus secretion, increased signs of eosinophils in bronchial fluid, and chronic inflammation.

Asthma is divided into multiple categories based on the type of symptoms that are being experienced. These include exercise-induced asthma, allergic asthma, and non-atopic asthma. The most common type of asthma is non-atopic.

Asthma has been linked to poor dietary habits as well as viral respiratory infections. Exposure to viruses that cause upper respiratory infections, such as rhinovirus, may precede an attack or flare-up in asthmatics. These infections cause an inflammatory response and release of cytokines that result in a state of asthma.

Symptoms

A person with asthma may experience various symptoms that can be divided into three categories:

• Shortness of breath: This symptom is characterized by immediate, recurring, and sudden exacerbations of airway constriction. Shortness of breath occurs due to both hyperactivity and spasm in the airways. This can result in wheezing and coughing, which may cause individuals to cough up mucus accompanied by chest pain.

• Breathlessness: This symptom is characterized by periods of prolonged breathing where exertion or physical activity typically cause individuals to breathe rapidly or pant. After exercise, asthmatics are left with feeling exhausted or fatigued and shortness of breath.

• Coughing: Individuals with asthma may experience a cough accompanied by chest pain or mild wheezing. The cough is generally associated with coughing up mucus, which can be associated with chest pain.

Treatment

Doctors believe that there are two primary factors that contribute to an asthmatic attack or flare-up. These factors include triggering factors and underlying risk factors. Triggers that can cause an asthmatic attack include cold air, exercise, allergies, and infections such as respiratory tract infections or the common cold. Those who develop asthma due to infection should consult their physician regarding treatment options prior to experiencing a trigger-induced flare-up.

While there are multiple treatments for asthma, the goal is to avoid triggers that may result in an attack or flare-up. Some of these triggers include avoiding tobacco smoke, dust, animal dander, strong air fresheners, and cleaning chemicals. It is also important to note that the use of fireplaces in homes can be dangerous as they can cause asphyxiation. Using a humidifier may help relieve symptoms associated with dry air; however, it is essential to clean the unit regularly to prevent mold growth.

Psoriasis

Psoriasis is an immune-mediated inflammatory condition that causes the skin to become red, itchy, and scaly. In addition, psoriasis can lead to symptoms such as joint pain, weakness, and fatigue. Psoriasis affects approximately 3 million Americans and is believed to be the most common autoimmune disease in the United States. It tends to occur more commonly in individuals of European or Asian descent, with the highest prevalence occurring among individuals of Ashkenazi Jewish descent.

Symptoms

There are three different sets of symptoms that may result from psoriasis:

• Generalized, symmetric erythema: This symptom is characterized by spread-like patches of redness on the skin. The red skin may sometimes appear thick and shiny as a result of the increased production of skin cells that build up on the outer layer.

• Erythrodermic psoriasis: Erythrodermic psoriasis causes the same symptoms as generalized psoriasis; however, it also causes symptoms such as fever, fatigue, and weight loss.

• Scalp psoriasis: Scalp psoriasis is characterized by dry, scaly patches on the skin followed by cracking and lesions.

Treatment

There is a wide range of treatment options for those who have been diagnosed with psoriasis, including topical ointments, ultraviolet light therapy, daily multivitamins, and immunosuppressants. Some individuals may also benefit from oral medications such as methotrexate.Due to the wide array of treatment options, it is important for a person to consult with their physician prior to selecting a specific course of treatment, especially if the individual has multiple locations of psoriasis.

Crohn's disease

This is a persistent inflammatory condition affecting the digestive system. The ileum, or lower part of the small intestine, is generally affected, although it can also travel upward and impact other areas of the digestive tract. Individuals diagnosed with Crohn's disease may experience physical symptoms such as abdominal pain, diarrhea, and fever.

Most individuals diagnosed with Crohn's disease will experience two or more symptoms at some point during their life. The typical age range for an individual diagnosed with Crohn's is between 15 and 45 years old.

Symptoms

The most common symptom associated with Crohn's disease is abdominal pain, which may be either cramping or sharp pains that last one to two hours. Additional symptoms associated with Crohn's disease include diarrhea, fatigue, and skin rashes.

Treatment

There are many treatment options for individuals diagnosed with Crohn's disease. Treatment may include oral medications or surgery to remove portions of the gastrointestinal tract.

If an individual experiences severe cases of Crohn's disease, they may require additional medications to limit the immune response within the body and reduce symptoms such as abdominal pain and diarrhea.

Eosinophilic esophagitis

Eosinophilic esophagitis is a disorder that involves an inflamed and excessively populated esophagus with an abnormally high number of eosinophils. The inflammation may cause symptoms such as chest pain, difficulty swallowing, or reflux.

Eosinophilic esophagitis is most common in children, with an estimated incidence of over 60 new cases in every 100,000 individuals per year.

Symptoms

The most common symptom associated with eosinophilic esophagitis is chest pain or dysphagia (difficulty swallowing). Additional symptoms associated with eosinophilic esophagitis include a lump within the pharynx (throat), heartburn, and regurgitation.

Treatment

There is a wide range of treatment options for those diagnosed with eosinophilic esophagitis. Treatment options may include the use of oral steroids and antibiotics or daily medication to reduce inflammation within the esophagus.

Some individuals may also benefit from adding a liquid form of foods or special diets to their diet.

Ulcerative colitis

This is a condition of the colon that causes long-term inflammation and ulceration in your bowel wall. It typically occurs in individuals with a family history of inflammatory bowel disease and individuals who have undergone prior surgery or may have an underlying condition known as UC-associated colitis. The inflammation of the colon causes symptoms such as abdominal pain, diarrhea, and fever.

It is believed that individuals with this condition can develop Crohn's disease. Approximately 30% of those diagnosed with ulcerative colitis may experience complications such as liver failure, extraintestinal manifestations (causing symptoms outside the colon), or cancer. Individuals with ulcerative colitis are at a greater risk for colorectal cancer due to the inflammatory nature of the condition.

Symptoms

The most common symptom associated with ulcerative colitis is abdominal pain, which may be described as cramping or intense pain within the abdominal region. Additional symptoms include diarrhea, fatigue, and fever.

Treatment

There is a wide range of treatment options for those diagnosed with ulcerative colitis. Treatment options may include the use of oral medications or daily medication to reduce inflammation within the colon. Additional treatment options include surgical procedures, steroid injections, and dietary changes such as the addition of fiber to the diet.

Lupus

Lupus, more commonly known as lupus erythematosus, is a chronic inflammatory disease of the skin and various organs in the body. It can result in many symptoms like pain, fatigue, and joint pain, as well as organ-related problems like arthritis and seizures.

The severity of symptoms varies on an individual basis. Approximately 0.3% of the total population is diagnosed with lupus, with women being twice as likely to be diagnosed as men.

Symptoms

The most common symptom associated with lupus is a skin rash, which may be described as red or purple spots on the skin. Additional symptoms associated with lupus include joint pain and muscle pain throughout the body.

Additionally, individuals diagnosed with lupus may experience headaches, fatigue, and difficulty breathing due to lung irritation or congestion.

Treatment

There is a wide range of treatment options for those diagnosed with lupus. Treatment options may include oral medications or daily medication to reduce inflammation within the body. Additional treatment options include physical therapy and steroid medications.

Lupus is an ongoing condition, and as an individual, as lupus ages, there is a greater risk of developing additional symptoms.

Possible treatments for inflammation

There are many different possible treatments that may be used to relieve inflammation within the body. The most common treatments are:

Dietary approaches

The diet plays a vital role in reducing inflammation within the body. Many individuals benefit from reducing their dietary intake of saturated fats, added sugar, and processed foods in order to reduce inflammation.

How does the diet help treat inflammation? Dietary approaches work by altering how the body metabolizes food. An individual may benefit from eliminating foods such as dairy products and refined carbohydrates to reduce inflammation. A diet high in fiber, found in fruits and vegetables, encourages healthy digestion.

Fiber also boosts the immune system and can slow down the formation of fats that put individuals at risk for inflammation.

2. Medication: It is often necessary to use medication to relieve inflammation. Common medication options for inflammation vary depending on the underlying condition that causes inflammation. A person should consult a health professional before taking medication. The medication options include:

OTC medication

OTC medication is an oral medication that can be used to relieve symptoms of inflammation. Examples of OTC medication options include Advil, Aleve, Tylenol, Motrin, and the like.

Nonsteroidal Anti-Inflammatory Drugs (NSAIDs)

NSAIDs medication are helpful in reducing inflammation. Ibuprofen (Motrin, Advil), naproxen (Aleve, Aleve-D), and aspirin are examples of common NSAIDs. NSAIDs may have negative effects on those with heart disease, high blood pressure, and asthma. Aspirin may be used in those individuals with underlying health conditions who take small doses.

However, individuals should consult a health professional before taking this medication option. The use of NSAIDs may increase the risk of bleeding in those with bleeding disorders.

Some individuals do not respond well to NSAIDs due to side effects or because a person is at an increased risk of developing gastrointestinal bleeding from the medication. Pataday and Voltaren eye drops are administered directly into the eyes to reduce inflammation.

These medications may be helpful in avoiding the stomach upset that is caused by some of the over-the-counter medications. A health professional should be consulted prior to using these medications. These medications also have potential side effects that include blurry vision, increased eye pressure, and headaches.

Acetaminophen

Acetaminophen is a medication that reduces inflammation by lowering the production of prostaglandins. This medication may be considered an option for treating arthritis and some other inflammatory conditions. Some individuals experience liver damage when taken or administered through injection, so acetaminophen should only be used for short periods.

Individuals who use acetaminophen for prolonged periods may experience loss of appetite and weight loss. Individuals taking other medications containing acetaminophen should be careful not to double dose. A health professional should be consulted prior to using these medications.

Prescription Medication

Prescription medication may be used to treat inflammation. The most common options are corticosteroids, biological response modifiers, immunosuppressants, and other medications that suppress the immune system, such as Remicade, Humira, Enbrel, and Cimzia.

A health professional should be consulted prior to using these medications.

Immunosuppressants

Immunosuppressant medications are drugs that put a person at an increased risk for infection. They include Etanercept (Enbrel), and Infliximab (Remicade). The medications are commonly used to treat arthritis and other inflammatory conditions such as Crohn's disease or psoriasis.

These medications are likely to cause side effects and may lower the ability to fight infections. Individuals who use immunosuppressants or steroids for prolonged periods are at an increased risk of developing an infection.

A health professional should be consulted prior to using these medications.

Intrauterine Devices (IUDs)

A wide range of intrauterine devices can be used to reduce inflammation. The most common types used include Mirena and ParaGard. IUDs may be used to treat irregular or heavy menstrual bleeding, endometriosis, uterine fibroids, and cancer.

A health professional should be consulted before using these types of devices.

Corticosteroids

Corticosteroids are a class of medication that can be used to reduce inflammation. Corticosteroids are available in pill form or in an injectable form (Cortisone) that may be administered through the skin. These medications come with side effects and are recommended to be used for a short period.

Side effects include headaches, mood changes, nausea, and muscle loss. Long-term use of corticosteroids may put individuals at an increased risk of developing diabetes or osteoporosis. A health professional should be consulted prior to using these medications.

Prescription NSAIDs

Prescription NSAIDs are a class of medication that can be used to reduce inflammation. Prescription NSAIDs include Celebrex, Mobic, Naprelan, and Oxaprozin. These medications should not be taken by individuals who have inflammatory conditions of the stomach or small intestine, ulcers, or take anticoagulant medication.

Individuals who take prescription NSAIDs for more than two weeks are at an increased risk for gastrointestinal bleeding. A health professional should be consulted prior to using these medications.

Exercise

Routine workouts are vital in reducing the possibility of chronic inflammation. Physical activity improves cardiovascular health and helps keep individuals free of heart disease. Regular exercise helps build muscle and boosts the immune system.

Individuals who participate in regular physical activity are less likely to develop cardiovascular disease and type II diabetes, which can both lead to inflammation. Exercising on a regular basis may take an individual out of the sedentary lifestyle that increases the risk for cardiovascular disease.

Supplements

Taking vitamins and supplements may help reduce inflammation. Vitamin B6, folate, etc., play a vital role and offer potent anti-inflammatory benefits. In addition to reducing inflammation, individuals who regularly take these supplements are less likely to develop chronic diseases such as cardiovascular disease and cancer. Common supplements include:

• Magnesium: The body uses magnesium to control inflammation, and it has the potential to lower cholesterol levels. Some studies have shown that magnesium may be a good dietary supplement for those who have high cholesterol.

• Vitamins D, C, and E: Vitamin D and E can potentially lower inflammation. Vitamin C may reduce the response to injuries on cell walls.

• Curcumin: Curcumin is a powerful anti-inflammatory ingredient that can be found in turmeric and has the potential to lower inflammation.

• Omega 3s: eg. DHA and EPA. Omega 3s have the capability to minimize inflammation and lower the chances of developing cardiovascular disease, cancer, and other age-related diseases.

Chapter 3: Types of Anti-Inflammatory Diet

Different diets can be used to assist in the treatment of inflammation. The possible diets used to treat inflammation include vegan, vegetarian, South Beach, and Mediterranean diets. These specific diets may reduce inflammation. Individuals should consult a health professional before changing their diet due to possible food allergies and other medical conditions. There are three types of Anti-Inflammatory diet are:

Mediterranean diet

Nuts, legumes, whole grains, fruits, and vegetables make up the Mediterranean diet. Red meat and fatty foods are prohibited on the Mediterranean diet.

Benefits of a Mediterranean diet

• Research shows that the four variables which are generally found in a Mediterranean diet do not only prevent heart disease but also reduce blood pressure, help you lose weight if you're overweight, and prevent stroke.

• The Mediterranean diet decreases your risk for metabolic syndrome: Research suggests that the combination of fish, nuts, and olive oil in the Mediterranean diet may combat metabolic syndrome. It is thought that this combination is what aids in lowering your risk for diabetes and cardiovascular disease.

• Reduces Women's Risk of Stroke: Research suggests that the Mediterranean diet may reduce a woman's risk of stroke. What's more, this diet may also help protect women against cardiovascular disease. Also, cases of cardiac diseases in women can be minimized by following a Mediterranean diet that includes foods such as olive oil, nuts, fruits, and vegetables.

• Prevents Alzheimer's Disease: Those who follow the Mediterranean diet are at a reduced chance of suffering from cognitive decline diseases. Research suggests that the antioxidants found in olive oil may be what protects those who follow this diet from developing Alzheimer's.

• May Stave Off Type 2 Diabetes: Research suggests that those who follow a Mediterranean diet are at a reduced risk of developing type 2 diabetes. Individuals should not completely eliminate carbohydrates from their diets and should consider all type of foods.

• Some Foods in the Mediterranean Diet May Ease Depression: Those who follow the Mediterranean diet are at reduced risk for depression. One of the main components of this diet is fish, which has been shown to increase good cholesterol (HDL), which can improve your mood.

• Supports healthy blood sugar levels: The Mediterranean diet helps keep blood sugar stable because of the high portion of healthy fats and low glycemic index foods. The healthy fats in nuts, olive oil, and fish can stabilize blood sugar levels.

• Protects the functionality of the brain: Studies show that omega-3 fatty acids found in fish may support brain function and prevent dementia. Dementia is a group of symptoms that affect the mental abilities of a person, such as forgetfulness and difficulty thinking, judging or communicating. The fatty acids found in fish may help those with dementia live healthier lives.

What foods should you eat on a Mediterranean diet?

You should base your diet on these healthy Mediterranean foods:

• Vegetables: The main portion of the Mediterranean diet is vegetables. Carrots, broccoli, and onions are all beneficial to your health.

• Fruits: You should eat a variety of fruits to keep your body healthy. The most important fruit that you should eat is peaches, which help prevent breast cancer and Alzheimer's disease.

• Nuts: Nuts are healthy foods that you should include in the Mediterranean diet plan. The most important nuts in this diet are almonds, walnuts, and pistachios, which have all been shown to lower cholesterol and protect against heart disease.

• Legumes: Beans and lentils are essential to your Mediterranean diet plan. These legumes are high in fiber and help you lose weight by keeping you full.

• Fish: The fish you eat should be as fresh as possible. Salmon, tuna, herring, and anchovies are all fish that should be part of the Mediterranean diet.

• Poultry: You should also eat poultry. Poultry is a healthy source of protein.

• Eggs: The eggs that you eat should be free-range and organic. Adding more eggs to your diet can help lower your cholesterol and may support a healthy immune system. It is okay to eat two eggs every day; you should not eat more than two yolks per day; you can eat egg whites, but try not to eat more than two egg yolks.

• Dairy: Dairy is the main ingredient in meals. The best dairy products to eat are low-fat or non-fat milk, yogurt, and cheese.

• Herbs and spices: You should use herbs and spices when cooking. The most important herbs and spices are oregano, sage, thyme, and rosemary, as they positively affect your immune system.

• Healthy fats: Healthy fats should be a part of your diet. Olive oils, canola, and peanut oils are the essential oils you should eat. You should also eat nuts, seeds, avocados, fish, and egg yolks.

Foods to limit

These processed foods should be limited in the Mediterranean diet:

• Refined grains: Whole grains are a healthier alternative to refined grains. Whole wheat products, brown rice, and oats are all healthy foods that you can eat in your Mediterranean diet.

• Trans fats: Trans fats shouldn't be used in cooking. These fats are unhealthy and should be avoided.

• Refined oils: Refined oils are a high-calorie ingredient that should be used only in small quantity. You should not use them as a part of your main diet.

• Processed meat: Processed meat contains high calories; they are unhealthy and should be removed from your diet. Processed meat includes hot dogs and sausages; all are high in sodium and fats.

• Highly processed foods: Highly processed foods can be a contributor to high cholesterol, obesity, and heart disease. Highly processed foods include store-bought cookies, cakes, and desserts.

Beverages

Water is essential in a Mediterranean diet. Every diet should include plenty of water. Tea and coffee are also good for you; just make sure to avoid sugar and milk.

Coffee and tea are also healthy beverage choices. Be mindful of added sugar or cream. Try to stick with quality tea brands, such as Traditional Medicinal, which use only organic herbs.

Healthy snacks

The Mediterranean diet is not just about what you eat at mealtimes. Almost any food can be a healthy snack. Here are some snacks to include in your diet:

• A handful of nuts.

• Olives.

• A piece of fruit.

• A bowl of yogurt with berries.

• A handful of mixed nuts and seeds.

• A small handful of dried fruit and almonds or walnuts.

• A few slices of cooked beets, carrots, or sweet potato (without added fat).

• Small amount of cheese cubes or fresh mozzarella balls (without added fat).

• Fresh vegetables with hummus dip (made from chickpeas, lemon juice, and olive oil).

Low sugar diet

This involves reducing added intake of sugar. This type of diet is effective for controlling blood sugar levels, reversing insulin resistance, and preventing or treating diabetes. A moderate-sugar diet improves diabetes while lowering cholesterol and preventing cardiovascular diseases, several malignancies (including breast cancer), and fatty liver disease.

Because it doesn't require eliminating all foods that contain sugar, a low-sugar diet is easier to follow than a no-sugar diet. This dietary plan can aid in developing a more healthy and balanced eating pattern by increasing your awareness of how much sugar you consume each day.

Benefits

• Reduced cholesterol: The diet can lower bad cholesterol levels in your blood, which is linked with an increased possibility of developing cardiovascular diseases. This is because a high intake of sugary foods can lead to an imbalance in your body's production of cholesterol, and the consumption of sugary foods and beverages can increase these levels

• Less abdominal fat: A low-sugar diet can help you lose weight by helping you to control your appetite and eat fewer calories. The low-calorie content of foods makes it easier to achieve this and reduces some of the strain that a high-calorie, lower-fat diet can put on your body.

• Reduced risk for serious diseases: A low-sugar diet can reduce your risk of developing serious conditions linked to diabetes, including type 2 diabetes and heart disease. This is because high levels of glucose, an excess of which is referred to as hyperglycemia, can lead to inflammation and oxidative stress in the body, which cause damage to cells and tissues.

• Fewer cravings: A low-sugar diet can help reduce cravings for sugar. Sugar addiction is a disturbance in the brain's reward circuit, which occurs when people consume high levels of sugar, causing dopamine levels to drop. This leads to a feeling of depression and anxiety, which can make a person crave more sugar.

• Healthier skin: A low-sugar diet can help keep your skin looking younger, as it may reduce the need for higher levels of vitamin C.

• Better sleep: A low-sugar diet can help you sleep better, as it can reduce the body's release of cortisol, which correlates with increased sleep disturbances. Adequate sleep can improve your health and reduce the chances of diseases.

• Improved mental health: A low-sugar diet can help improve your mood, as it may reduce levels of the stress hormone cortisol. This is because a low-sugar diet helps to increase levels of neurotrophic factor (BDNF), the protein responsible for regulating learning and memory functions.

What foods should you eat?

The following foods are recommended for a low-sugar diet:

• Leafy green vegetables: Broccoli, spinach, kale, and other leafy greens are all excellent sources of vitamins A and C, iron, folic acid, and fiber.

• Fruits: Lemons, limes, oranges, and berries are all excellent sources of vitamin C. They can be eaten in small amounts to help with weight control.

• Whole grains: Oats, brown rice, pearl barley, and quinoa are all whole grains endowed with high fiber concentrates. They play a role in managing sugar levels in the blood, reducing your chances of developing diabetes.

• Beans and legumes: Beans and legumes are low in fat and protein and an excellent fiber source. They can help to control blood sugar levels.

• Sweet potatoes: Sweet potatoes contain vitamin A plus other antioxidants, which can help to control levels of sugar in the blood.

• Nuts and seeds: these are excellent sources of fiber and can help to slow down the digestion of carbohydrates, helping you feel fuller for longer.

• Fatty fish: They can lower inflammation and lower the chance of developing heart disease.

• Lean proteins: they contain a variety of nutrients that minimize the chances of cardiac disease and type 2 diabetes. Examples of lean proteins are eggs and chicken.

Foods to avoid

• White bread or flour: White flour is made from processed wheat, which has been stripped of most of its nutrients. It may contain added sugar, leading to an increased risk of diabetes and obesity.

• Refined sugars: Refined sugars, usually in the form of soft drinks and desserts, contain added sugars. They are a hidden source of sugar that can cause chronic inflammation and weight gain.

• Sugary drinks: Soft beverages contain a high level of calories and whole sugar and should be avoided.

• Packaged snack foods: Packaged snacks are high in fat and sugar. Although they may contain reduced-fat or fat-free versions of foods, these healthy changes are often not made, especially when the food is aimed at children.

• Alcohol: Alcohol can negatively impact your blood sugar levels, which can lead to changes in appetite and mood.

Is the low-sugar diet a healthy choice for you?

If your main aim is to lose weight and improve your health, a low-sugar diet will assist you in achieving these goals. If you are overweight or obese, the low-sugar diet is a healthy choice, as it is low in calories and can help you lose weight. If you have an existing health condition such as heart disease or diabetes, this diet will help eliminate these issues by reducing inflammation and oxidative stress.

Health benefits

• Reduced risk of type 2 diabetes: A low-sugar diet helps in managing glucose levels in the blood, thus reducing the possibility of having type 2 diabetes.

• Reduced risk of heart disease: This diet improves your cholesterol levels, hence eliminating your chances of having coronary artery disease and cardiac arrest.

• Reduced inflammation: It reduces the harmful effects of inflammation on blood vessels and the immune system. This is because a low-sugar diet helps to improve insulin function and glucose tolerance, which reduces chronic inflammation in the body.

• Reduced oxidative stress: A low-sugar diet helps lower oxidative stress markers, which can protect you against disease. This is because a low-sugar diet can help reduce saturated fat intake and protect you against harmful free radicals in your body.

• Reduced risk of obesity: It reduces the fatty amounts your body stores and increases the amount of fat your body burns, which can reduce the chance of you becoming overweight or obese.

• Improved mood: A low-sugar diet may improve your mood, as it can positively affect levels of certain neurotransmitters in the brain, including serotonin.

Health risks

The low-sugar diet can also be too restrictive for some people's tastes. Is the low-sugar diet healthy for you?

If you have diabetes or a health condition that is affected by blood sugar levels, and you don't follow the diet correctly, it may be too dangerous for your health to follow this diet plan. The low-sugar diet may not be suitable for people with a sweet tooth or those who like foods containing added sugars.

Pescatarian diet

The fat content in a pescatarian diet is low, but the protein content is high. This is because fish provides a considerable amount of the necessary vitamins, minerals, and fatty acids the body needs.

Benefits of a pescatarian diet

• Improved cardiovascular health: This plan is a good choice for those with high cholesterol levels as it can help reduce their bad (LDL) cholesterol, lowering their risk of cardiovascular disease.

• Improved overall health: A pescatarian diet will help to improve your overall health as it is rich in vitamins and minerals, which are essential for the body's healthy functions.

• Weight loss: A pescatarian diet can help you to lose weight by reducing your calorie intake and increasing the amount of exercise you do, which will help to burn calories.

• Healthy pregnancy: A pescatarian diet is a good choice for pregnant women, as it is high in nutrients and protein. It provides the right amount of vitamins and minerals to meet a baby's needs during growth and development.

• Healthy baby: A pescatarian diet is also healthy for babies, as it helps to meet their nutritional requirements so that they can grow up to be strong and healthy.

A pescatarian is someone who is a vegetarian who occasionally eats fish. The word "pescatarian" has its origin from the Latin word Pesce, meaning fish. The word "vegetarian" is derived from the Latin word vegus, meaning whole edible plants. Pescetarian meals can be simple to prepare.

A good source of protein is seafood (fish). Other sources of protein are found in nuts, beans, and legumes. Seafood is a great way to get healthy fats without consuming too many calories. Many species, such as salmon, mackerel, and tuna, are rich in omega-3 fats.

Vegetarians who have decided not to eat meat can be at risk for developing a deficiency of vitamin B-12 if they don't plan their diet properly. A healthy nervous system and the production of red blood cell function are both made possible by vitamin B-12. The finest food sources of vitamin B-12 include dairy, chicken, and eggs. By consuming these foods, pescatarians can get the needed amount of B-12 each day.

Steps for being a pescatarian

1. Find out about the different types of fish that you can eat: Tuna, salmon, and sardines are examples of fish that contain omega-3 fats, which can help people with high cholesterol levels lower their bad (LDL) cholesterol. Other types of fish, such as flounder and tilapia, may not be as healthy. They are low in omega-3 fats but high in saturated fat.

2. Read the nutritional information on seafood packages: Seafood that has been farmed is not as healthy because they have had its natural fish oils stripped away.

3. Learn how to prepare seafood: Use common sense when handling unfamiliar fish such as tuna, and salmon. The most common way of cooking is by broiling or roasting. Steaks and fillets should be cooked over high heat quickly for about three minutes and then turned over or basted with cooking oil during cooking to prevent the flesh from drying out.

4. Plan your meals: Make seafood, egg, and dairy-based dishes the main components of your diet. You can choose healthy options from any day of the week.

5. Buy fish in bulk packages from a retailer you trust and make sure it is fresh before cooking: The freshness of seafood should be one of the most important things to consider when buying fish because it could affect how healthy and tasty the dish is going to be.

6. Mix it up: Variety is the spice of life, so keep trying different seafood. You will find healthy ways to include fish in your diet that you never thought possible.

7. Take a vitamin B12 supplement or eat foods that are fortified with B12: While the body of a pescatarian can meet the RDA for vitamin B12 with minimal effort, vegetarians have to make an effort to find a source of this vitamin in their diet because they do not consume any foods from animals and since Vitamin B-12 is found only in animal products. Some vegetarians take a vitamin B12 supplement.

8. Be active: you will have to exercise in order to keep your weight down. In order to burn fat more efficiently during exercise, the body needs more protein than carbohydrates; thus, consuming protein after a workout will help you rest more comfortably as your body repairs itself post-workout.

9. Drink less: Consuming a lot of white sugar, soda, and other sugary drinks can lead to weight gain. You should limit your intake of sugary drinks to about one or two daily (one for breakfast and a couple for an afternoon snack).

10. Watch your portion sizes: A pescatarian needs to be mindful of their food intake for the above reasons. Be aware of how much you eat and ensure that every bite contributes to your overall dietary plan. Don't be afraid to have this as part of your meal plan; it is perfectly normal!

11. Stay focused and stick to your diet: Changing your dietary habits to include more seafood and less meat will make you at least an 80% pescetarian.

Why do people choose a pescatarian diet?

People choose a pescatarian diet for many reasons. Many people choose a pescatarian diet for ethical reasons. Some people don't want to consume any animal flesh. Others are not comfortable with the potential cruelty involved in the dairy and egg industries or are worried about the environmental damage that large-scale animal farming can cause.

Some pescatarians choose it as a healthier alternative to other diets; some even do it because they don't want to be restricted by following a vegetarian or vegan lifestyle. Consumers can make choices that are right for them without feeling as though they have to adhere to a specific diet.

Issues with being a pescatarian

Some people who follow a pescatarian diet choose not to consume any animal product, including dairy and eggs (vegan). Being a vegan is more difficult than being a pescatarian since the vegan has many more restrictions placed upon him or her. Vegan diets are often lacking in calcium, vitamin D, and vitamin B12. Some voluntary vegetarians will still consume dairy products or eggs but not meat.

The same concerns about calcium, vitamin D, and vitamin B12 apply to these types of vegetarians as well. Another issue that may be brought up is that many non-meat eaters have a different opinion of pescatarians than they do of vegetarians and vegans. Although pescatarians and vegans will often gladly share the idea of being compassionate to animals, many people are skeptical about the ability to be fully committed to the cause.

Some people make this choice for ethical reasons and find it easier to adhere strictly to a pescatarian way of eating no matter what other people think. Anyone who follows these dietary guidelines must be aware of the possible health risks that can come with it. There is evidence that people who consume fewer animal products have a reduced risk of cancer, but higher intakes are linked with higher chances of cancer and cardiac diseases.

Pescatarians definitely face a challenge when it comes to getting enough protein daily and consuming the right amount of fat for their body type. If dieters do not plan their meals correctly, they may be at risk for developing cases of malnutrition. As with any diet, it is important to consider all aspects of health, including mental as well as physical health, when choosing how you want your diet to look and feel.

What should you eat?

• Whole grains and grain products: bread, pasta, rice, cereal, etc. Whole grains are good for the body as they are full of fiber, which helps digestion. They also provide additional vitamins and minerals that can benefit an overall healthy diet.

• Legumes and their products: Legumes are also very important for healthy pescatarian diets. They are a very good source of protein and fiber. Legumes can be used for various dishes, and many people who follow the pescatarian lifestyle will try to incorporate them into their meals as much as possible. Some examples include lentils, beans, split peas, peanuts, soybeans, and peanut butter.

• Nuts and nut butter: Almonds, cashews, peanuts, and walnuts are great examples of nuts that can be used in pescatarian diets. Nutritionally nuts are extremely good for people and will help them to get all the nutrition they need.

• Dairy: Pescatarians can eat dairy items such as milk, cheese, and yogurt.

• Eggs: While fish is generally considered a pescatarian's primary source of protein, people who follow this diet can still consume eggs as well as other foods that contain high levels of protein. Eggs contain vitamins such as A and B, minerals, and electrolytes.

• Fruits: Fruits are rich in some nutrients that are extremely important for healthy bodies. They contain large amounts of potassium and folic acid. Fruits such as apples, pears, strawberries, oranges, and bananas provide pescatarians with all the nutrition they need while following a diet.

• Vegetables: Vegetables like broccoli, cauliflower, and lettuce are very good for a person's health. They are high in fiber and other minerals, which helps in running the body smoothly. A vegetable diet will help pescatarians stay healthy without worrying about missing out on any nutrients they need.

Foods that pescatarians don't eat

• Beef: Beef is widely consumed due to its high protein content, which has earned it the title of a"' superfood.'" However, this doesn't mean that everyone can consume it. People who have allergies to beef or people who choose not to eat meat for ethical reasons are not allowed to eat this type of meat.

• Pork: Similar to beef, pork is another meat that contains a lot of protein but also contains high cholesterol levels and should be avoided by anyone who doesn't want to harm their health.

• Chicken: Based on the type of protein that chicken contains, they are not fit for consumption by the pescatarians.

• Lamb: While lamb isn't as popular as other meats, it too contains a lot of cholesterol and should be avoided.

• Turkey: Although turkey isn't very popular in the U.S., it is often eaten by Japanese people as they consume it quite often because of its health benefits.

Chapter 4: Preparing for a Healthy Diet Lifestyle

This is the way of life that makes it possible to stay in shape and live a more fulfilling life. Everyone should try to achieve a healthy lifestyle by staying fit and leading a happy lifestyle. It can be easy to follow if one knows what they are looking for. There are a number of steps one needs to take in order to make it work:

Correct mindset

The mindset is important. Being convinced that one can live a healthier lifestyle while eating the foods one wants is key. It needs to be clear that one should not use dieting as an excuse to eat less and/or unhealthy food; rather, it should be viewed as an opportunity to expose their body to the right kinds of food.

Exposing your body to the right kinds of food means that it will be getting everything that it needs to function better. If you decide to work out and eat a healthy diet, you will notice many changes in your body, such as better moods and less risk of getting sick. The mindset will also help one remain determined throughout the process.

No good or bad food

Another aspect of the mindset one has to have is that there are no bad or good foods; they are all just foods. This is an important point because having this mindset will help you eat every kind of food and avoid feeling guilty about it as well as avoiding any diet mentality. For every certain food, there are always certain benefits to it that might be interesting to know, such as a fennel seed salad might help one lose weight faster, while a banana can have many health benefits.

One might also have to think about the foods they eat and how they can be prepared, whether by adding a little vinegar or seasoning them with different spices. This will help one enjoy the right kinds of food while also being able to do so in a healthy way. It is also important to understand that there is no right way to eat. Just as every person has their own taste, they will eat differently depending on their social group.

Eat mindfully

This is a good practice and will help you stay in shape. Eating mindfully means slowing down and focusing on every bite you take. It also means enjoying all your food's tastes, textures, and smells. This way of eating can be done at any time. It could be done after work or even before going to bed, where there are only a few things that need to be done for it to be successful. It helps one feel better about their health, social group, and immediate environments.

Keep it realistic

No one should be under the impression that they will lose ten pounds in one week by eating a certain way. It can be frustrating to have unrealistic expectations of what the process will be like. If you are serious about losing weight and improving your health, making small daily changes is better. A great way to do this is by keeping a food diary or chart where you can track how many calories you eat each day and also what you eat for each meal.

By tracking this amount, you can see how many calories you take in and how much exercise you do. You can then see the difference between how much you eat and how much you burn. This will make it easier to improve from there. This way, you will be able to make a positive contribution to your health by eating better and exercising more. It should also be kept in mind that it is not whether or not you lose weight that matters but rather how much effort you put forward in making the changes that happen in your life.

How much better do you feel emotionally and physically when following a healthy diet, and how it helps you in lowering your inflammation? Your primary focus should be to live a healthy lifestyle, which will help you lower inflammation.

Making home cooking less inflammatory

Cooking at home is a great way to cook your meals and eat the way you want to eat. The food you cook at home gives you a greater sense of being in control of your health. Cooking at home is also cost-efficient, saves time, and makes it easy for you to follow what you really want to do in terms of eating habits.

When it comes to cooking at home, one needs to be mindful of what they are eating because many foods can have certain inflammatory properties. Inflammation can be caused by the consumption of meat injected with hormones, along with the consumption of fried foods containing oils and fats.

The food that one can cook at home is the kind of food that does not have those properties. It can be homemade cakes, stews, vegetable-based meals, etc. Meat and fish that are consumed at home should be cooked properly. They should not be burned so much or overcooked because both of these will cause the meat to have an inflammatory effect on one's body

Taking it one meal at a time

This is another important aspect of eating out of one's mind. One needs to be consistent with what he is doing in terms of his diet and exercise regimen. If one doesn't eat properly, it will not make much difference in how fit one is. If one decides to exercise, exercising for 30 minutes every day will not make much difference if the person does not eat the right kind of foods.

Tips to prepare for a diet change

Like any other lifestyle change, the initial period is filled with uncertainty and doubts as to whether it will benefit you. It is important to be realistic about what it will take to become successful in your goals. The idea behind making a change in your diet is that a person feels better about himself; that way, he will be able to do things he would not have done otherwise. With this being said, there are things that people can do in order to prepare themselves for this kind of change. Some of the things that people can do include:

1. Don't shop without a list: People often shop out of impulse and end up with all sorts of unhealthy food in their refrigerators. You must have a list of what you need before you go shopping so that you do not buy things that are not on the list and end up eating them later. This way, the healthiest option is the one that you will have to eat.

2. Replace your favorite "junk" food restaurant: You should consider changing or even looking for a healthier alternative. This way, instead of eating at a restaurant that gives you unhealthy options, you can instead replace it with something healthier.

3. Glycemic index and high glycemic foods: The glycemic index denotes the rate at which a specific food is digested and absorbed in your body. It depends on various factors like the speed of the vegetable or fruit turning into sugar, e.g., carrots, potatoes, and beets turns into sugar faster than beans or whole grains. Look up the glycemic index of foods you are going to eat and find out how they will affect your blood sugar levels so that you can keep them under control while dieting.

4. Try a new healthy recipe once a week: It is important to find a healthy recipe that you can make on a regular basis. If you like to try new things, you can combine vegetables, fish, and chicken with whole grains and legumes in order to make a meal. You can also try adding some nuts or seeds to your meal.

This way, you will learn to cook new things and make your meals interesting. Finding a new recipe is important because you will, on most occasions, stick with the dietary plan when you are being creative by adding new things to your meal each week. Also, when you are trying something new and want to learn how to cook it, you will make sure that you use the right ingredients for the dish.

5. Cook more often: Eating at home rather than going to restaurants is a great way to maintain weight. This way, you will be in control of what you eat and how much you eat. This is a great way to avoid unnecessary expenditure on food as well. When you are at home, you know exactly what goes into your food, and the ingredients you use are fresh.

Cooking at home will help keep your body healthy and fit by eating more nutritious food. Most of the dishes served in restaurants contain unhealthy ingredients that you should be avoided. Also, when you cook at home, you will be more likely to eat at regular intervals because of the time that it takes to cook. Eating at regular intervals ensures that you do not overeat because of hunger.

6. Become more active: Exercise is a great way to lose weight. You can go for morning walks, run or jog after work, swim, dance, etc. Some people love to exercise while they are following a healthy diet because they have more energy and feel healthier. There is a saying that goes, "You are what you eat," meaning that weight and fat are determined by the food we put in our bodies.

If you go for cardio and strength training, your body will work harder, and you will see results faster. Doing cardio and strength training is a great way to stay away from the cravings and temptations of unhealthy food.

7. Proper Sleep: This is very important for everyone. You will be more likely to overeat if you are not getting a good night's sleep. You should go to bed and get up at the same time every day so that your body clock can adjust accordingly. If you get a good night's sleep, your metabolic rate will increase, which means that you will burn calories faster.

Taking enough rest will also help to put you into a relaxed state where you can avoid the stress that often leads to overeating. Being stressed will make you want to eat unhealthy things. Also, if you are a person who struggles with stress, it can be quite difficult to go through diet changes because of the stress that it causes you. To avoid overeating during this time, try going for a walk or other forms of exercise and relaxation.

8. Know which foods are good choices: It is crucial to figure out which foods will contribute positively to lowering your inflammation and also will help you in fat loss. You can do this by reading up on different kinds of diet plans. An internet search will lead you to quite a few diet plans, but you can also visit the library and read books on the subject.

Also, google the types of diet plans you are thinking of trying and learn more about them in order for you to make a wise decision on what kind of plan you want to follow for yourself. You should also check up on the plan you will be following every once in a while because newer versions of the same diets and guidelines might come out.

9. Call restaurants for questions or to review their menu: If you are on a diet and go to a restaurant, you should ask the waiter how they prepare their food. If it seems like they are using ingredients that are not healthy, then you should avoid eating at that restaurant because these might put you in danger of overeating.

When you eat out, ask the waiter how much quantities of certain items cost so that you can order accordingly. Avoid going to restaurants that serve beverages that are not healthy, and check out their menu before going there. If they have many unhealthy options on their menu, you should avoid eating at that restaurant because you will be at risk of overeating and eating the wrong things. A restaurant that doesn't offer healthy options is not worth it because you might end up spending a lot of money on food that does not help your anti inflammation goals.

10. Pay attention to serving size: It is very common for people to get the wrong idea about how much food constitutes a serving size. For example, when cooking rice, try keeping the cup of rice that you will serve yourself at home separate from the amount of rice you eat at restaurants. This way, you will know for sure what a serving size of rice is, and it will help you control your portions if you take some time to prepare your meals in advance.

This way, you will be able to have more control over how much food you eat and how often. Also, purchasing a food scale to measure the amount of food you eat is a good idea. This will be helpful if you are on a diet where your intake of calories is measured.

11. Watch for hidden sources of unhealthy ingredients: You should carefully monitor the ingredients in your food. This way, you will be able to avoid unhealthy foods and ingredients. It is important that you go through what ingredients are used in the foods you eat every day to know what foods are healthy and which aren't.

If a restaurant uses many unhealthy ingredients, you should seriously consider avoiding it. Also, look for hidden sources of trans fats in the foods you purchase so you do not consume trans fats.

Supplements that fight inflammation

Research shows that supplements can be used to fight inflammation. The pain, tenderness, and swelling that comes with inflammation can make it hard to perform your daily activities. Supplements may help alleviate some of the symptoms while reducing the underlying issue that is causing the inflammation. The following are some excellent supplements to help relieve the discomfort caused by inflammation:

1. Curcumin is an orange pigment found in Mother of Pearl and other vegetables such as turmeric, ginger, and beets. Curcumin has anti-inflammatory properties and is effective at reducing pain due to inflammation. Good sources include turmeric root, ginger root, and black pepper extract. You can purchase curcumin in supplement form at most vitamin stores.

2. Fish oil: A recent discovery found that people have little or insufficient fatty acids in their food. These fatty acids are needed to fight inflammation, and they can also help decrease heart disease. If you are unable to get enough omega-3 in your diet, you may need to supplement your intake of fish oil. Fish oil is used by many athletes and elderly people who have difficulty getting the right nutrients in their diets.

Fish oil supplements have not been proven effective for arthritis; however, many users find relief with the added anti-inflammatory properties. You can purchase fish oil capsules at most vitamin stores or grocery stores.

3. Ginger: Ginger is a strong anti-inflammatory. The anti-inflammatory properties of ginger are also drawn from its essential oils, which have anti-viral and antimicrobial properties. Ginger is used to treat many pain conditions. Good sources include fresh ginger root and powder extract. You can purchase fresh ground ginger root at most grocery stores and spice stores. Good sources also include ginger extracts found in most multivitamins or vitamin supplements.

4. Resveratrol: Resveratrol is a phytoestrogen that can be found in plants such as grapes, blueberries, peanuts, and soy. Resveratrol inhibits the enzymes used by some cancers to grow. Resveratrol also has anti-inflammatory properties and can be found in multiple weight loss supplements as well as some anti-aging products. Resveratrol is also good at lowering blood pressure and reducing cholesterol. You can purchase resveratrol in pill form at most vitamin stores or online.

5. Spirulina: Spirulina is a type of blue-green algae cultivated in bodies of water around the world. Spirulina has a good amount of protein and can be acquired in powder form at many health facilities or pharmacies. Spirulina has many healing properties, including reducing inflammation, boosting the immune system, and fighting viruses and bacteria. You can purchase spirulina at most health food stores or vitamin supplement stores.

6. Vitamin D: this is a fat-soluble vitamin that can be found in foods such as salmon, tuna, and eggs. Vitamin D is also produced in the body by the sun. Vitamin D plays a large role in fighting inflammation and reducing pain. Vitamin D can be found in pill form at most health food stores or pharmacies. You can also visit your doctor to be tested to determine if you are deficient in vitamin D.

7. Bromelain: Bromelain can be found in pork. It is also used as a meat tenderizer. Bromelain works by reducing swelling and boosting the immune system. Bromelain can be bought in pill form at many health facilities or veterinary offices. It is not effective for all types of pain, but it can be very helpful for relief from arthritis-related pain.

8. Green tea extract: this is very common in many weight reduction supplements and is also effective at fighting inflammation. Green tea contains antioxidants and polyphenols that fight the underlying causes of chronic pain. You can purchase green tea extract in pill form at most vitamin stores, although most weight loss supplements will contain the active ingredients found in green tea.

9. Garlic: Garlic contains anti-inflammatory properties that reduce joints' swelling. Garlic can be purchased in pill form at most vitamin stores, but it can also be found in many spice racks across the country. Fresh garlic and garlic powder are both effective at reducing inflammation and pain.

10. Vitamin C: Vitamin C is an excellent anti-inflammatory and can be found in foods such as citrus fruits, tomatoes, and bell peppers. Many non-steroidal anti-inflammatories also cause weight loss by reducing appetite and increasing metabolism. You can purchase vitamin C tablets in pill form at most vitamin stores or grocery stores.

Keeping your cool when dining out

Dining out is a great way to try new foods and explore the flavors of different culture. But eating out can expose you to harmful bacteria, which can cause gut inflammation. While these restaurants may not appear dirty, they often use poorly handled or contaminated ingredients. If you suffer from inflammatory diseases and want to safeguard your health while dining out, here are a few tips and tricks to help you keep your cool during your meal.

1. Consider a vegetarian diet or avoid red meat

A study by the American Journal of Preventive Medicine found that vegetarians were 48 percent less likely to develop inflammatory bowel disease than their meat-eating peers. So if you are looking for an anti-inflammatory diet, try substituting red meat for fish and chicken as much as possible.

2. Go for organic eggs and dairy products

Organic eggs are rich in Omega-3 fatty acids, a surefire way to keep your inflammation low. Furthermore, organic eggs are free from harmful antibiotics, hormones, and chemical additives found in conventional eggs. The same can be said for dairy products. Conventional milk and cheese products often contain added antibiotics and growth hormones that will certainly exacerbate inflammation in your body.

3. Avoid junk food and processed foods

Junk foods are loaded with harmful fats and additives that only exacerbate inflammation in your body. Processed foods, such as packaged snacks, candy, frozen meals, and cookies, are better at increasing inflammation than fresh fruits and vegetables.

Another reason to avoid these foods is that they are often high in sodium, which will cause you to retain water weight. Also, consulting a nutritionist is highly recommended when dealing with inflammatory diseases such as arthritis or psoriasis.

4. Cut out trans fats

Trans fats will increase inflammation in your blood and body. They are found in many processed foods, but not all fried foods. The best way to avoid trans fats is to purchase the label "hydrogenated oil" on your food packaging and avoid the oils used for cooking, such as canola and corn oil.

5. Avoid high fructose corn syrup

High intakes are linked to increased body inflammation. It is found in most processed foods; keep a keen eye out on any food packaging to avoid this product.

6. Cut out sugars and alcohol

Sugar will spike your blood glucose levels, causing insulin resistance. The same goes for alcohol, which will also increase inflammation in your body.

7. Steer clear of dairy products

Many people are unaware that most cases of inflammatory bowel disease are due to a sensitivity to dairy products. The Journal of the American Medical Association found that people who consume an average of five or more servings of dairy daily have a 1.4 to 2.8 times increased risk of developing inflammatory bowel disease.

If you suffer from inflammatory bowel disease and want to protect yourself, always check the label on your dairy products to confirm if there are any casein, lactose, and lactobacilli, which are the main culprits for increasing inflammation in your body.

8. Limit your intake of alcohol

If you are looking for a way to keep your inflammation low, you should limit the amount of alcohol you consume. This is especially true for those who are prone to inflammation. Alcohol will significantly increase inflammation in your body by increasing the production of stress hormones and reducing levels of anti-inflammatory hormones. Not only that, but alcohol calories should also be considered as they can contribute to weight gain.

If you are at a buffet, it is a good idea to tell the server what you can and cannot eat. If a dish contains something that you cannot eat, do not touch it or get near it.

Importance of fats

Getting enough fats into your diet is essential for maintaining a healthy weight. Fat is important for your health because it is a necessary dietary nutrient. However, not all fats are created equal. It is important to distinguish between the fatty acids and other types of fats found in foods.

There are many different types of fat depending on their molecular structure (what they are made up of). Fats that come from animal products tend to be long-chain polyunsaturated fats (LCPUFA), while plant-based oils are mostly composed of saturated fatty acids (SFAs).

The more unsaturated fat a food has, the less likely it is to cause inflammation. There are two types of unsaturated fats: monounsaturated and polyunsaturated. The type of LCPUFA in fat also determines how easily it can be metabolized and if it will clog up your arteries.

Omega-6 FFA is found most commonly in animal products (meat, eggs, fish), while omega-3 FFA is found primarily in plant oils (flaxseeds, walnuts, soybeans, and canola oil).

Human and animal studies have shown that omega-3 FFA has many benefits for maintaining health and preventing disease. For instance, they can raise the good (HDL) and reduce the bad (LDL) cholesterol levels in your blood.

Additionally, omega-3 FFA has been demonstrated to reduce inflammation and benefit those who suffer from chronic diseases.

Other research has demonstrated that omega-3 FFA can improve mental function and treat conditions, including depression and ADHD. Heart disease may be avoided with the aid of omega-3 FFA.

They can lower blood pressure, relieve congestive heart failure symptoms, reduce triglycerides, and delay the artery plaque buildup that could result in a heart attack or stroke.

Fats are also a very important part of the diet for healthy skin and hair and to maintain a healthy weight. Only small amounts of fats are required for these functions, but it is still very important to maintain a healthy omega-6 to omega-3 ratio in the diet.

The ratio plays a significant role in whether or not you will develop inflammation in your body.

The ideal ratio is 1:1, which means that there are about equal amounts of omega-6 and omega-3 FFA in this diet. These foods are composed of; flaxseeds, walnuts, soybeans, and canola oil. Omega-6 fatty acids are present in most foods in the form of linoleic acid.

In addition to animal products such as meat and eggs, omega-6 fatty acids can also be found in plant oils. For example, corn oil contains 157 mg of omega-6 FFA per one tbsp (14 g)

Two important factors determining fat's health benefits are how easily the body metabolizes it and how much it is saturated. In general, unsaturated fats are easier for the body to break down and use than saturated fats, which the body cannot use very well.

Monounsaturated and polyunsaturated fats are more easily metabolized in your body than saturated fat.

Tips to achieve lasting change

In order for a change to be effective, it has to be sustainable. The following tips will help you achieve lasting change in your diet:

1. Adopt a new eating style. You will have to change your normal food intake, your eating routine, and the quantity you eat.

2. Form healthy habits. Habit formation is the key to making lasting change. It's easier to be healthy when you don't have to think about it and can do it automatically. Identify the specific triggers that are causing inflammation.

Then avoid them to stop the inflammatory response. Some common triggers include food, medications, emotions, pain, and pollution. When you form a habit of avoiding these triggers, you'll reduce inflammation throughout your body.

3. Make changes gradually. If you try to change too much at once, you will probably be overwhelmed by the task and give up before you even get started.

4. Be flexible with your plan, but do not stray too far from it. It is important to set a plan and stick to it as much as possible in order to see results. The key is balance. There are plenty of foods you can enjoy while also eating healthier foods regularly; this way, when you indulge in a treat, it will not be so bad for your body compared to if you never compromised with yourself and always ate healthy snacks or meals only.

5. Set realistic goals for yourself. You should have specific and measurable goals for your change. Make sure that you are clear about what goals you have for yourself.

6. Practice portion control when eating out or drinking alcohol. Since you will be consuming more foods over time, your intake will likely increase as well. Make sure to measure the portions you receive at restaurants and bars (if it is not already on the menu) so you know what to expect.

7. Keep track of your progress daily (or at least a few times weekly). This is an excellent way to keep yourself on track. You will be more likely to see gradual change if you are aware of it, which will help you continue your plan.

8. Reward yourself for your hard work at the end of every week or month. Do not reward yourself with food, though! Think of something that will not jeopardize your success (for example, shopping for new clothes that are smaller than what you are now).

Chapter 5: Deciphering Anti-Inflammatory Nutrition

Anti-inflammatory nutrition is the way to go for many people, but it is not always easy to determine which foods are the "best" choices. The key is choosing a diet that you can easily keep up with. If you do not eat certain foods regularly, you most likely can not make up for the lack of intake of special nutrients. Here are a few tips on making your anti-inflammatory diet satisfying and easy to follow:

1. Fill your plate to fight inflammation

Eat plenty of fruits and vegetables. There are many studies that have shown that eating lots of different fruits and vegetables reduces and prevents inflammation in the body. The types of fruits and vegetables that will give you the most health benefits include berries, apples, sweet potatoes, bananas, and leafy green vegetables.

2. Make the right diet choice for you

Be aware of your diet and the foods you eat regularly. Choose anti-inflammatory foods that you will keep up with for an extended period. Remember, inflammation has many causes and can be controlled in more than just one way. A balanced, healthy diet is the most effective treatment for chronic pain and arthritis disorders.

3. Conquer carbs

If you are trying to reduce your carbohydrate intake, do so slowly. Try reducing carbohydrates by 10% each week and then monitor the effects. Remember that not all carbs are bad; in fact, some are actually beneficial.

4. Get the right protein

Making sure you get the right amount of protein is key to a healthy diet. Knowing where to look for proteins without large amounts of unhealthy fats can be difficult. Try choosing grass-fed meat, fish, eggs, and legumes to get the right amount of protein with healthy fats and few calories.

5. Indulge in sweets

If you are trying to reduce inflammation in your body, it is probably a good strategy to avoid large amounts of sugar and sweets. However, this does not mean that you can't enjoy some treats every now and then. Portion out your treats so that it is not too much for one meal.

How to design your new personal food and lifestyle

This is a personal plan designed specifically for you. It is based on your current lifestyle and the foods you have been eating regularly. If you want to help your body maintain healthy joint structures and improve mobility, then a diet made up of foods with low inflammation and inflammation-fighting nutrients can be very helpful.

The diet that you select should be able to deliver these nutrients while also making your lifestyle enjoyable and convenient. Try to work with a nutritionist or registered dietitian who can help you determine the right foods based on your nutrition needs and your life situation.

Here are some suggestions that may help you design your new personal food plan:

1. Avoid inflammatory foods: Many foods have been identified as promoting inflammation in the body. The following are specific examples of foods that should be avoided or eaten in moderation:

• Fried foods
• Foods high in saturated fats, such as processed food items and pork products
• Red meats and processed meats
• Excess sugar, salt, and trans fats (found in processed foods)

2. Eat plenty of whole grains every day: Whole grains are very important to a healthy diet. They provide energy for your body, keep blood sugar levels steady, and offer a number of nutrients. The following are some examples of whole grains that you can consume:

• 100% whole wheat (bread, pasta, and crackers)
• Steel-cut oats
• Brown rice

3. Choose anti-inflammatory fruits and vegetables every day: Fresh fruits and vegetables are great sources of many important nutrients. They also can help to reduce inflammation. Some examples of anti-inflammatory fruits and vegetables include:

• Leafy greens, such as spinach and kale
• Berries, such as raspberries and blueberries

4. Incorporate healthy fats into your diet daily: Healthy fats are good for your body because they help improve the function of your cell membranes (found in every cell in your body). They also help to produce many important hormones. While it is important to consume healthy fats, special attention should be paid to the source, as not all types of fats are created equal. Here are some examples of healthy fats that you can include in your diet:

• Nuts, such as almonds, walnuts, and peanuts
• Seeds, such as pumpkin and sunflower seeds
• Avocado (natural fat found in avocado) • Natural oils found in olive oil (extra-virgin olive oil) and avocados

5. Take advantage of spices: Fresh spices such as onion, garlic, and fresh ginger can help support a healthy immune system without creating high amounts of inflammation. Spices are also easy to add to almost any food to boost flavor and nutrients. Here are examples of spices that you can use in your diet:

• Turmeric (root)
• Lemon (juice)
• Cayenne pepper

6. Drink plenty of water each day: Staying hydrated is important for many reasons, especially if you want to support a healthy immune system. Drinking water also helps to regulate digestion, balance your body temperature, and even helps to reduce stress.

7. Make exercise fun: Exercise is important in helping the body maintain its proper structure and function. However, it can be boring and tedious. When adding exercise routines into your daily life, try to make them fun and easy to follow so that you will be more likely to stick with them for an extended period of time. Don't forget that exercise also has another benefit: it helps to reduce stress levels by releasing endorphins into the body.

8. Don't forget about your mental health: It is important for you to remember that you are not just your body. Your spirit and mind are important, too. Make sure that you take time each day to relax and de-stress without feeling guilty or lazy. There are many ways to reduce stress, such as a warm bubble bath, a good book, or music. If you have days when everything is going wrong, take a deep breath and try to look at the big picture to find peace in the bigger picture of life.

9. Have fun: Take some time each week to do something just for fun. This will help to keep you from feeling stressed and burnt out. Some examples of fun things that you can try include:

• Enjoy a lazy afternoon with friends and family or alone with a good movie

• Try a new activity that you have never tried before, such as quilting, scrapbooking, painting, or baking

10. Make healthy eating sustainable over the long term: It is important for you to remember that it takes time for your body to heal itself. Your new habits should be sustainable over the long term so that they don't become too overwhelming to maintain. For example, you may get your new habits started by:

• Setting a goal to lose 10 pounds over the next few months and then continue to monitor the results

• Making small changes, such as substituting one junk food for an equivalent healthy alternative daily

• Determining how long it takes for these small changes to add up to your goal weight, then deciding if you are ready to make any additional changes.

11. Be patient and follow through: While it is easy to get discouraged and give up when things don't go quite the way you had hoped, persistence is key to achieving your long-term goals. You should have a plan in mind to be successful so that you can make it through the first few difficult days. Use rewards for yourself each week so that you are more likely to stick with your new program.

12. Don't forget about life outside of your new lifestyle: Don't lose sight of your goals and how they will affect other aspects of your life. If you feel like skipping a few workouts because you are tired, feeling sick, or noticing that your clothes aren't fitting quite right, remember that you are worth it, and don't stop when life gets in the way. Instead, make the changes to fit all aspects of your life.

Enjoying your health and wellness will spill over into other areas of your life, including family time and work. Think about how much better you will feel when you are full of energy and have more stamina to play with your kids or excel at work. This positive outlook will help motivate you to continue the process even if it doesn't seem realistic initially. Try to focus on the long term instead of the short term.

13. Get support: Surround yourself with positive people instead of negative individuals who will only make you feel worse about your goals. Reach out to friends, family members, or a fitness professional if you need help or encouragement while working on your new lifestyle changes.

When choosing a fitness professional to help you with your nutrition for healthy weight loss goals, you should choose someone who can provide both nutritional counseling and exercise guidance. This is the best way to get the most out of your efforts and make the process easier.

14. Make healthy eating a lifestyle: Healthy eating does not have to be a temporary experiment or diet. You should make healthy eating part of your life so that you are more likely to remain successful in achieving your goals. Choose healthy food options, such as whole grains and fresh fruits and vegetables, instead of processed foods with added sugars, trans fats, and calories from fat.

15. Stay motivated and consistent: While motivation is key for any diet, it is even more important when trying to achieve your weight loss goals. To stay motivated over the long term, set small, intermediate, and long-term goals. These goals should be a consistent routine that fits into your lifestyle instead of an occasional fad diet.

16. Be realistic and plan: Don't start a diet you can't stick with. If you want to start exercising every day, make sure that you know that you can do it before starting, or else you are likely to give up along the way when things get harder than they first seem. Eat healthier foods gradually instead of eliminating all junk food immediately.

17. Don't be afraid: Your fears keep you from being successful in anything, so it is important to overcome your fears by training yourself to overcome the challenges you face.

18. Don't skip meals: Skipping meals is not part of a healthy eating routine. Make sure you eat enough to function and stay energized throughout the day. Don't let your busy schedule or other commitments interfere with your meal planning.

19. Choose smaller plates: This simple trick can help some people eat healthier. When you use smaller plates to eat your meals, you are more likely to fill up on healthy foods without overeating. It is important to choose a meal plan and eating style that works for you to avoid feeling deprived or hungry.

20. Experiment with new things: Don't be shy or afraid to try new food choices if they are part of a healthy lifestyle. You should never feel like you are missing out on anything because there are always substitutes for cravings of unhealthy foods or food portions. Make sure you don't fall back into the old routine because the substitutes taste good!

Action plan

Once you have read through the tips above and incorporated them into your daily lifestyle, we suggest you to complete the action plan below. This should take roughly two weeks so that your body gets used to the changes and begins to get rid of extra weight.

Set small goals that are easily accomplished:

• Try to set 3-5 small goals each week by working towards completing small tasks instead of trying to accomplish too much in one day. These tasks can include anything from eating at a few different healthy restaurants to consuming only one caffeinated drink each day while not drinking any other beverage.

• Once you have set your goals, try to follow them daily. Make it your goal to always try to do this. You will eventually be more likely to succeed because your body will become accustomed to following through with tasks that you have set for yourself.

Plan out your meals:

• Plan out at least four healthy meals a day. Make sure you are getting all the nutrients your body needs by eating small amounts of fruit, vegetables, lean meats and fish, beans/legumes, and whole grains throughout the day.

• Plan out three healthy snacks a day. Try to choose between fruits, vegetables, protein shakes, or a combination of other snack foods that are healthy and available to you. You should look for meals high in fiber when possible so your digestive system can get the nutrients it needs daily.

Plan for cheat meals:

• Plan out your cheat meals. If you eat at a restaurant once a week without changing anything else in your eating habits, this is considered cheating. You should plan out this meal and what you will order instead of allowing yourself to be tempted by food choices that are unhealthy for you.

Set goals that take into account your lifestyle:

• Although some people find it helpful to stick with the same meal plan or set of meals daily, most people need flexibility. This is important because shifts in your lifestyle can interfere with your ability to stay on track. For example, if you live in a cold climate that restricts your outdoor activities over the winter months, it will be important to change your meal plan so that you can eat more regularly indoors.

The same is true if you often travel during vacations or are going through a difficult time. If you know that your schedule is going to change frequently and you are planning to eat healthy at these times, then try a meal plan with flexible options that allow for modifications in portions so that you don't feel deprived when special occasions arise.

Pantry stock

It is important to buy ingredients you will need to complete your meal plans and snacks. You should first purchase a variety of meats, fish, and produce so that you can taste your way around the kitchen and find foods you enjoy. You should choose three fresh, healthy fruits per day:

• Choose a mixture of foods that contains both fruit and vegetables. You should avoid eating a single vegetable as the main component of your diet. You must try out many variations to find what works best for you.

Again, these guidelines can be used to plan out the first month or two of your healthy eating plan. You will be able to find your solutions along the way, but knowing what works for others can get you started on your path toward finding success in healthier eating for weight loss.

Tips

Once you have read through the tips in this book and come up with a plan ideal for your lifestyle, you can find out more ways to help yourself fight inflammation. Remember that every body is different and what works for some people will not work for others:

1. Keep a journal of how often and why you eat junk food and other information about your eating habits. This will be helpful once you start making healthier food choices because you can see where there are opportunities to improve your diet even more.

2. Store healthy snacks in areas that are inaccessible. This helps prevent eating junk food when you are in between meals. It also prevents tempted unhealthy snacking.

3. Make better choices when choosing what and how much to eat by having healthy foods with you at all times. Game time snacks and healthy foods should be at the top of your list.

4. Eat when you are hungry and stop eating when you are full, but avoid snacking on junk foods between meals. As mentioned above, this is referred to as "changing your mindset" about what and how much to eat.

5. Choose foods that promote satiety: Satiety is the feeling of being full. Certain foods can make you feel fuller for a longer period than others. These include fruits and vegetables, beans/legumes, and whole grains.

6. Avoid trigger foods: This is when you eat something unhealthy because the food tastes good or reminds you of something else you liked in the past. These foods include processed and fatty foods and sweets. Trigger foods are usually the reason that you typically eat junk food.

Benefits of stopping inflammation in its tracks

It is no secret that inflammation can lead to many health problems, including diabetes, cancer, heart disease, and more. So what are the benefits of stopping inflammation?

1. Happier mood: Eliminating inflammation will greatly improve your mood and make you happier. You can lift those dark clouds of depression and anxiety by simply changing your lifestyle.

2. Sharp brain: Many anti-inflammatory foods contain antioxidants that improve memory. These include berries, nuts, olive oil, and dark chocolate. Your memory will improve, and you will notice a big difference in how quickly you can process information.

3. Low risk of heart and cardiovascular disease: Reducing inflammation will reduce your risk of heart disease and stroke. The bad news is that enlisting a healthcare professional's help is not something you should take lightly. Each office will have a different opinion, and you must consider the pros and cons of each.

Considering your health history, finding out what foods you can eat and how these choices work for you is critical in helping you find your best weight-loss plan. An alternative to choosing a dietician or nutritionist as a primary resource would be to use forums like askjeeves.com, which allow people with similar questions to find answers from other people who have been there and found success in healthy eating.

4. Decreased cholesterol levels: You may also choose to go on a cholesterol-lowering regime, which will require you to follow a special diet. In addition, you should exercise at least 30 minutes per day to promote good blood circulation, which is crucial for insulin production and blood movement through your body.

5. Decreased risk of diabetes and metabolic syndrome: Any diet plan to lose weight should also be combined with diabetes and metabolic syndrome treatment plan. You should choose foods low in sugar but high in fiber, such as whole-grain cereals, legumes, and bread. Be careful not to eat too much fat because this can lead to weight gain.

6. Weight loss is the obvious benefit of changing your lifestyle. Changing your diet and exercise habits will lead to weight loss, improve your health and give you the confidence you need to be at a healthy weight. Choosing a healthy lifestyle is the key to successful weight loss and management.

7. Strong bones: If you add strength training to your workouts, you can lose weight and increase your bone density. Strong bones will help to prevent osteoporosis, one of the big health problems in America that are caused by weak bones.

8. Decreased risk of autoimmune disorders: Inflammation plays a big role in autoimmunity, which can cause chronic health problems such as fatigue, insomnia, joint pain, and cognitive decline. A healthy diet will also help prevent these autoimmune disorders by lowering inflammation levels in the body.

9. Lower risk of cancer: Recent research clearly illuminates that a diet rich in anti-inflammatory nutrients can reduce risks of cancer, including cancers of the colon, lung, breast, pancreas, and prostate. Many of these foods are also anti-cancer agents. In addition to removing inflammation from your diet plan, you may take supplements or use guided meditation or music to be more mindful to help control inflammation levels in your body.

10. Improved fertility: Inflammation can lead to autoimmune disorders and fertility problems. This can be especially a problem for women trying to get pregnant. If you are trying to get pregnant, you should consider adding foods that have anti-inflammatory properties to your diet.

Conclusion

As you can see, inflammation can be a big problem. However, there are several steps you can take to stop inflammation and improve your overall health. The key is to consider your food choices, exercise habits, and lifestyle carefully to make the best decisions for yourself.

A healthy lifestyle requires a shift in thinking and a commitment to good health. Making changes to your diet and lifestyle will improve your health not only in the short term but also in the long run as well. The key is to be patient and not give up because it can take several weeks or even months for these changes to make a difference.

Exercising and eating healthy food are key to a healthy lifestyle. If you have an obesity problem, detoxification is a process you might consider kick-starting your weight loss efforts. It is not a diet but can help you make healthy lifestyle choices by helping you avoid foods that cause an immune response. It teaches you the benefits of eating anti-inflammatory foods that not only reduce inflammation levels in your body but may also help your body release toxins more efficiently. When these toxins are removed from the body, your immune system will function better and your overall health will get better.

Fats are necessary in your diet for a healthy heart and a robust central nervous system. Fatty acids, including Omega, are provided by eating foods rich in fat, such as avocados, nuts, and seeds. Eating plenty of fiber-rich fruits and vegetables is also important because they will help you feel full and stop you from craving foods that contain harmful ingredients that may cause an immune response.

Ultimately, following a diet plan will help you fight inflammation and improve your general health by preventing many diseases, such as cancer, diabetes, and heart disease.

Your mindset is critical to losing weight. People who look in the mirror and dislike their appearance may feel bad about themselves. This can cause them to eat more than they should and make unhealthy lifestyle choices. When you start feeling this way, you need to remind yourself that your body is not the enemy-your body is a temple, and you are in charge of it.

Your mind and emotions play a big role in how you feel about your body, so try to be mindful of what is going on in your mind. Inflammation can cause pain, headaches, and other nagging symptoms in the body. Try making more positive choices to limit stress, anger, and fear. These emotions can wreak havoc on your health and lead to many chronic health conditions.

Having enough sleep is paramount to good health. Poor sleep can lead to inflammation and other chronic health problems. When stressed, try to unwind by taking a shower, having a hot tub, listening to music, or getting some fresh air with nature. Your body needs time to regenerate at night and will be more receptive to physical activity in the morning.

Your diet is a big part of your success in losing weight and improving your overall health. If you want to make changes that last long-term, you must follow your diet plan no matter how uncomfortable it might be because life will get much easier in the end if you stay on track with what you are doing.

One of the keys is to eat healthy, anti-inflammatory foods. You can find many foods in your local health food store or supermarket. Many are rich in nutrients and other omega-3 acids, which enable our bodies to heal and reduce swelling. If you are concerned about making all the right changes, seek a nutritionist or diet planner to help you devise a diet plan that meets your unique needs.

It is important to continue exercising to be healthy and lean. Aerobic exercise such as walking can help you burn calories while building muscle strength that will improve your overall health and appearance. Strength training exercises, such as weight lifting, can also help by increasing muscle mass. It is also important to stretch and do yoga. Yoga calms the mind and body, relieves stress, and may help with joint pain. Being healthy is not difficult if you make the right choices for yourself.

Anti-inflammatory diets make it easy to lose weight and improve your overall health. It is not as difficult as you think and can be a healthy lifestyle choice. Sticking with the diet plan is tricky because you may have to cut back on certain foods that used to be a major part of your diet. If you stick with the plan, you will soon see the results for yourself, and it will be worth it.

Making changes to your lifestyle is hard work, but the rewards are well worth it. You will see your body change in a positive way that is both attractive and healthy. Your mind will also become clearer and more focused because of these changes.

You should not be afraid to change your diet to lose weight or improve your overall health. A healthy lifestyle is more than just losing weight; it is about making healthy choices that will benefit you in the long run, no matter your age. The key is to have a positive outlook on yourself and be kind to the body you have inherited.

Make sure you eat the foods your body needs and do not exercise if you are unwilling to put in some effort. You will begin seeing results almost immediately and will be glad you took the time to change. It's time to take charge of your health. You are not in this alone, and you can do it.Your health depends on it.

Recipes

Avocado Deviled Eggs

Servings-7, Kcal- 91, Proteins- 8g, Fats- 15g, Carbs- 1g

Ingredients

5-7 eggs
1 avocado
Salt (1/4 teaspoon)
Garlic   (1/4 teaspoon)
Pepper   (1/4 teaspoon)

Chilli   (1/4 teaspoon)
Paprika (1/4 teaspoon)
Cumin   (1/4 teaspoon)
Cilantro (2 tablespoon)

How to make Avocado Deviled Eggs?

First step is to boil the eggs. For boiling eggs, add eggs in a pot, then fill the pot with water, boil the water and let the eggs get boiled for 15- 20 minutes. After you have boiled the eggs, you need a bowl filled with cold water, using a spoon take out the eggs from hot water and put them gently in the cold water bowl.

Let the eggs cool down for a few minutes. Remove the shell. Cut the eggs in lengthwise shape and remove the yolk. Add all the spices and yolks to a bowl. Mix yolks and spices until they are combined. Now, place the mixture in egg halves. Top eggs halves with lime juice and cilantro.

Scrambled eggs

Servings-2, Kcal- 240, Proteins- 15g, Fats- 17g, Carbs- 1g

Ingredients

2 tablespoons of olive oil
4 egg whites

Salt, pepper and chilli

How to cook scrambled eggs

Take a medium bowl, crack the eggs in the bowl. Add salt, pepper, and chili. Whisk it well. Take a frying pan and heat olive oil. Now put the egg mixture in the pan and stir it well for few minutes and your eggs will be ready.

Kale & Coconut Shake

Servings-1, Kcal- 160, Proteins- 5g, Fats- 6g, Carbs- 13g

Ingredients

1 cup unsweetened almond milk
1/2 cup coconut milk
4 cups chopped kale
1 cup ice

1/4 cup ground coconut
1 1-inch piece fresh ginger
1/4 teaspoon kosher salt

How to make Kale & Coconut Shake

Combine all the ingredients in a blender and blend until smooth.

Green eggs

Servings-1, Kcal- 250, Proteins- 15g, Fats- 20g, Carbs- 4g

Ingredients

2 large eggs
2 leaves of kale

pinch of salt
1 teaspoon butter

How to cook green eggs

Place eggs, salt, and kale in a blender. Blend it till it becomes smooth. Heat oil in a frying pan and add egg mixture to the pan. Cook eggs for a few minutes. Your dish is ready to serve.

Salmon salad

Servings-2, Kcal- 450, Proteins- 30g, Fats- 34g, Carbs- 4g

Ingredients

½ cup walnuts
6 oz cooked salmon (small pieces)
6 cups of spinach
Salt

Pepper
2 teaspoons of vinegar
2 teaspoons of mustard
2 tablespoons of olive oil

How to make salmon salad

In a bowl, add mustard, vinegar, salt, pepper, and oil. Put greens on a plate and top with salmon and walnuts. Pour the dressing over and serve.

Feta, and olive salad

Servings-1, Kcal- 620, Proteins- 3g, Fats- 64g, Carbs- 3g

Ingredients

Pinch of oregano, dried thyme
2 tablespoons of olive oil
1 cup cucumber (chopped)

1 cup green olives
½ cup feta

How to make feta, olive and sundried tomato salad

In a large bowl add all the ingredients. Mix well. Serve.

Raspberry Macadamia Smoothie

Servings-1, Kcal- 550, Proteins- 28g, Fats- 15g, Carbs- 2g
Ingredients

4 tablespoons of macadamia nuts   Water
4 tablespoons of vanilla protein powder   ½ cup coconut milk
2 tablespoons of MCT oil   1 cup raspberries

How to make Raspberry Macadamia Smoothie

In a blender, mix all the ingredients. Blend well until smooth. Your smoothie is ready.

Scrambled eggs with spinach and feta

Servings-2, Kcal- 560, Proteins- 21g, Fats- 57g, Carbs- 1g

Ingredients

½ cup feta   6 cup spinach
8 egg whites   4 tablespoons of olive oil

How to cook scrambled eggs with spinach and feta

In a frying pan, heat oil at medium flame. Add spinach and cook until bright green (3 minutes approximately). Now add eggs and stir (2-4 minutes) until cooked. Now add feta and serve.

Strawberry Vanilla Smoothie

Servings-2, Kcal- 180, Proteins- 6g, Fats- 11g, Carbs- 8g

Ingredients

1/2 cup fresh or frozen strawberries

1/3 cup unsweetened coconut milk

2/3 cup water

1/2 teaspoon vanilla extract

How to make Keto Strawberry Vanilla Smoothie

Combine all the ingredients in a blender and blend until smooth.

Mean Green Matcha shake

Servings-1, Kcal- 334, Proteins- 19g, Fats- 24g, Carbs- 13g

Ingredients

1 cup almond milk

¼ cup coconut milk

1 scoop Vanilla Protein Powder

1 tablespoon coconut oil

1 scoop MCT Oil Powder

1 large handful spinach

1 small avocado

1 cup of ice (optional)

How to make Mean Green Matcha Protein Shake

Combine all the ingredients in a blender and blend until smooth.

Tropical Pink Smoothie

Servings-1, Kcal- 402, Proteins- 24g, Fats- 28g, Carbs- 12g

Ingredients

1/2 small dragon fruit
1 small wedge Galia
1/2 cup coconut milk
3-6 drops liquid Stevia extract

1 scoop vanilla protein powder
1 tablespoon chia seeds
1/2 cup water

How to make Low-Carb Tropical Pink Smoothie

Combine all the ingredients in a blender and blend until smooth.

Turkey Patties

Servings-1, Kcal- 240, Proteins-65g, Fats- 36g, Carbs- 3g

Ingredients

1 tablespoon olive oil
Salt
Pepper
1 egg

½ teaspoon sage
¼ onion
3/4 pounds turkey(without skin)

How to cook Turkey burgers with sage

Mix Salt, Pepper, 1 egg, ½ teaspoon sage, ¼ onion', 3/4 pound turkey and form into 2 patties. In a frypan heat oil and add patties, cook well on both sides for 5-8 minutes.

Shrimp fried rice

Servings-2, Kcal- 505, Proteins- 42g, Fats- 34g, Carbs- 3g

Ingredients

1 tablespoon sesame oil
½ tablespoon soy sauce
2 eggs (beaten)
½ pound shrimp (250 gram)

3 green onions
2 tablespoons of coconut oil
1 ½ cup cauliflower

How to cook shrimp fried rice

1. In a pan heat 1 tablespoon of coconut oil, add shrimp, and cook for 3-5 minutes. Remove from pan and set aside. Heat another tablespoon of coconut oil, add onions, and cauliflower.

2. Cook for 6 minutes approx. Add soy sauce and eggs to the pan and stir continuously. Add sesame oil and stir, then toss with shrimp and serve.

Roasted chicken thighs

Servings-3, Kcal- 573, Proteins- 105g, Fats- 15g, Carbs- 2g

Ingredients

2 pounds of boneless chicken thighs
1 tablespoon organic extra virgin olive oil
1 tablespoon chili powder
Sea salt to taste

ground pepper
fresh cilantro
lime wedges

How to make Chili roasted chicken thighs

Preheat the oven to 140 C degrees. Place the chicken on a baking sheet. Drizzle with olive oil and turn to coat. Rub with chili powder, salt and pepper. Roast the chicken legs in the oven for about 15 minutes. Sprinkle with coriander and serve with lime wedges.

Key Lime Pie Smoothie

Servings-1, Kcal- 281, Proteins- 8g, Fats- 22g, Carbs- 6g

Ingredients

1 cup of water

1/2 cup almond milk

1/4 cup of raw cashews

1 cup of spinach

2 tablespoons of shredded coconut

2 tablespoons of lime juice

How to make Key lime pie smoothie

Combine all the ingredients in a blender and blend until smooth.

Golden Coconut smoothie

Servings-2, Kcal- 460, Proteins- 24g, Fats- 30g, Carbs- 3g

Ingredients

2 tablespoons of MCT oil

4 tablespoons of vanilla protein powder

2 tablespoons of flax seeds (golden)

1 teaspoon turmeric

Water

1 and ½ cups of coconut milk

How to make Golden coconut smoothie

In a blender, mix all the ingredients. Blend well until smooth. Your smoothie is ready.

Chicken and Feta cheese plate

Servings-6, Kcal- 433, Proteins- 28g, Fats- 32g, Carbs- 3g

Ingredients

1 lb rotisserie chicken
1cup feta cheese
2 salt and pepper

10 black olives
1/3 cup olive oil
2 oz. lettuce

How to cook chicken and Feta cheese plate

Place chicken, feta, lettuce, and olives on a plate.

Season with salt and pepper as desired. Serve with olive oil.

Chicken bulgogi

Servings-1, Kcal- 650, Proteins- 50g, Fats- 30g, Carbs- 3g

Ingredients

3 tablespoons of avocado oil
1 chicken breast, cut into thin strips
1/2 medium onion, diced
3 tablespoons tamari sauce

1/2 tablespoon sesame oil
2 cloves of garlic, minced
Salt, to taste
1 teaspoon sesame seeds

How to cook Keto chicken bulgogi

Heat avocado oil in a large pan over medium heat. Add chicken and onion to the pan and fry until the chicken is cooked (about 5-7 minutes). Add tamari sauce or coconut aminos, sesame oil, and garlic to the pan and fry for about 1 minute. Season with salt and garnish with sesame seeds.

Tamari Chicken

Servings-2, Kcal- 500, Proteins- 80g, Fats- 13g, Carbs- 3g

Ingredients

1/4 cup (60 ml) avocado oil
1 lb (450 g) ground chicken
2 Tablespoons tamari sauce
Salt and pepper, to taste

1 Tablespoon fresh ginger
2 cloves of garlic (minced)
4 green onions, diced

How to cook Keto Tamari Chicken

Heat the avocado oil in a hot wok or pan. Add the ground chicken, green onions, garlic, and ginger. Fry until the meat is cooked. Add the tamari sauce and season with salt and pepper.

Chicken Hash Recipe

Servings-2, Kcal- 600, Proteins- 110g, Fats- 21g, Carbs- 3g

Ingredients

4 chicken breasts
1 medium onion, sliced
2 carrots, grated
Coconut Dijon sauce

1 leek, sliced
4 tablespoons coconut oil
Salt and pepper, to taste

How to cook Chicken Hash Recipe

Cook the diced chicken breast in coconut oil and fry until properly cooked. Season with salt and pepper as desired. If necessary, add more coconut oil to the pan and cook the vegetables gently. Add the chicken pieces back. Serve with Dijon coconut sauce.

Coconut Chicken Tenders

Servings-2, Kcal- 510, Proteins- 92g, Fats- 15g, Carbs- 7g

Ingredients

1 pound boneless chicken
1 egg
1/2 cup cashew flour
1 cup unsweetened shredded coconut

1/4 teaspoon salt
1/4 teaspoon pepper
1/4 teaspoon garlic powder
1/8 teaspoon of cinnamon

How to cook Coconut Chicken Tenders

Preheat the oven to 170 degrees C. Beat the egg in a bowl and set aside. Combine cashew flour, coconut, and spices in another bowl. Dip each chicken tender first in the egg and then in the batter

Place the coated chicken tenders on a baking sheet lined with aluminum foil or parchment paper. Bake for 15 to 20 minutes.

Easy coconut chicken

Servings-1, Kcal- 750, Proteins- 150g, Fats- 15g, Carbs- 4g

Ingredients

1 tablespoon coconut oil
5 cloves garlic
4 tablespoons of apple cider vinegar
1 lb boneless skinless, chicken thighs

1/2 teaspoon black pepper
1/2 teaspoon Sea Salt
1/4 cup water
1 cup coconut milk, canned

How to make Easy coconut chicken

Add the chicken and coconut oil in a large pan over medium / low heat. Cook for 2 to 3 minutes, then add apple cider vinegar, water, and cloves of garlic and cook for 3 minutes. Add salt and pepper and cook until all the liquid has evaporated.

This should take about 10 minutes. Stir in coconut milk and simmer for 5 to 10 minutes until the liquid has thickened slightly and you get a coconut mixture that looks like a sauce. Take off the stove and enjoy!

Easy Chicken + Spinach

Servings-4, Kcal- 550, Proteins- 120g, Fats- 10g, Carbs- 4g

Ingredients

2.5lb chicken
1 Medium Onion
1/2 pack of mushrooms
1/2 bag of frozen spinach
Salt + Pepper

1 Lemon
olive oil
Basil {dried or fresh}
Garlic Powder

How to make Easy Chicken + Spinach

Add oil to a large pan and then add your chopped onion and your mushrooms. Add your diced chicken to the pan, let it cook. When your chicken is almost ready, add basil, salt + pepper, and garlic powder to taste. Then add spinach. While cooking, add a little bit more oil and squeeze out the juice of a lemon. When your chicken is cooked and your spinach is heated, it's done!

Easy Mustard Chicken with Radish & Greens

Servings-1, Kcal- 700, Proteins- 150g, Fats- 11g, Carbs- 3g

Ingredients

1 tablespoon olive oil
3 tablespoons of yellow mustard
1 teaspoon garlic powder
1 cup radishes sliced

1 teaspoon salt
1 pound chicken breast raw
3 cups of collard greens chopped

How to cook Easy Mustard Chicken with Radish & Greens

Mix olive oil, mustard, garlic powder, and salt in a small mixing bowl. Brush the chicken breast with the mixture and marinate for at least 10 minutes. Heat a large pan over medium heat and add the marinated chicken breast. Let it cook for 10 minutes, then add radishes and collard greens. Stir regularly and cook for another 5 minutes so the green vegetables are properly cooked. Remove from heat and serve with salt to taste.

Chayote Chicken Noodle Soup

Servings-1, Kcal- 700, Proteins- 150g, Fats- 11g, Carbs- 5g

Ingredients

1 tablespoon olive oil
1/2 onion diced
6 cups of chicken broth
1 pound chicken pre-cooked
Salt and pepper to taste

1 cup water
1 teaspoon basil dried
1 teaspoon oregano dried
1 teaspoon parsley dried
2 chayote squash

How to make Chayote Chicken Noodle Soup

Heat oil in a large saucepan over medium heat. Add onion and celery, cook for about 5 minutes or until the onion becomes translucent. Add chicken broth, water, chicken, basil, oregano, parsley, salt, and pepper. Bring to a boil, then reduce the heat to medium, cover, and let simmer for 10 minutes. Cut the chayote squash into noodles with a spiralizer. As soon as the soup has simmered for 10 minutes, remove the lid and add chaya noodles. Simmer for another 10 minutes without the lid. Remove from the stove and serve.

Sardines and Onions

Servings-1, Kcal- 140, Proteins- 0g, Fats- 12g, Carbs- 2g

Ingredients

1 can (3.5 oz or 100 g) sardines in olive oil
1 teaspoon apple cider vinegar

Salt, to taste
1 tablespoon olive oil

1/4 red onion, thinly sliced

How to cook Keto Sardines and Onions

Place chopped onions in a bowl. Drizzle with vinegar and olive oil. Garnish with sardines. Sprinkle salt, as desired.

Scrambled eggs with smoked salmon

Servings-1, Kcal- 500, Proteins- 35g, Fats- 32g, Carbs- 3g

Ingredients

5 egg whites
2 tablespoons of avocado oil
50 g smoked salmon, chopped

Salt and black pepper to taste
1 teaspoon crushed peppercorns

How to cook Scrambled eggs with smoked salmon

Add 2 tablespoons of avocado oil in a pan over medium heat. Add egg whites into a bowl and pour into the pan. Scramble eggs slowly in the pan. Cut smoked salmon into small pieces and add them to the eggs before they cook.

Keep stirring until the eggs are firm - don't overcook. Place on a plate and season with sea salt, black pepper, and crushed pink peppercorns.

Salmon curry recipe

Servings-3, Kcal- 400, Proteins- 50g, Fats- 23g, Carbs- 3g

Ingredients

1/2 medium onion, diced
2 cups of green beans, diced
1.5 tablespoons of curry powder
1 teaspoon garlic powder
Cream from coconut milk

2 cups of broth
450 g raw salmon, diced
2 tablespoons of coconut oil
salt and pepper
2 tablespoons of basil

How to cook Salmon curry recipe

Fry diced onion in coconut oil until translucent. Add green beans and fry for few more minutes. Add broth or water and bring to a boil. Add curry powder, garlic, and salmon. Add coconut cream and simmer until the salmon is cooked (3-5 minutes). Garnish with salt, pepper, and chopped basil.

Salmon fish cakes

For salmon fish cakes –
Servings-8, Kcal- 177, Proteins- 20g, Fats- 8g, Carbs- 3g

Ingredients

3 cans of salmon
2 tablespoons of fresh dill
3 medium eggs, whisked
1/4 cup of coconut flour

1/4 cup of coconut oil (60 ml)
Salt and pepper, to taste
1/4 cup shredded coconut (20 g)
2 tablespoons of coconut oil

For creamy dill sauce –

1/4 cup of mayo
1/4 cup of coconut milk
2 cloves of garlic, minced or finely diced

Salt and pepper, to taste
2 teaspoons of fresh dill

How to cook Salmon fish cakes

Add all the ingredients of dill sauce in a small bowl. Mix properly. Combine the ingredients for the fish cake in a large bowl. Form the mixture into 8 patties. Melt 2 tablespoons (30 ml) of coconut oil in a large pan. Carefully place the patties in the oil. Cook golden brown on both sides for about 3 to 4 minutes. Serve the salmon patties with the creamy dill sauce.

Fried sardines recipe with olives

Servings-1, Kcal- 140, Proteins- 1g, Fats- 13g, Carbs- 3g

Ingredients

1 can sardines in olive oil
5 black olives, sliced
1 tablespoon garlic flakes

1 teaspoon parsley flakes
1 tablespoon olive oil

How to make Fried sardines recipe with olives

Add the tablespoon of olive oil to the frying pan and fry everything together for 5 minutes.

Mustard sardines salad recipe

Servings-1, Kcal- 130, Proteins- 1g, Fats- 12g, Carbs- 2g

Ingredients

1 can (4-5 oz) sardines in olive oil
1/4 cucumber, peeled and diced small
1 Tablespoon lemon juice

1/2 Tablespoon mustard
Salt and pepper to taste

How to cook Mustard sardines salad recipe

Drain olive oil from sardines. Mash the sardines. Combine sardines, cucumber cubes, lemon juice, mustard and salt & pepper. Mix well.

Tuna Stuffed Avocado Recipe

Servings-1, Kcal- 340, Proteins- 20g, Fats- 25g, Carbs- 3g

Ingredients

1 (5 oz.) can tuna
2 tablespoons greek yogurt
1 medium avocado (cut in half and pit removed)

pinch of dried dill
salt and pepper

How to make Tuna Stuffed Avocado Recipe

Combine tuna, Greek yogurt and dill in a small mixing bowl. Season it with salt and pepper as desired. Fill the avocado halves with tuna salad and serve.

Grilled Buttermilk Chicken

Servings-6, Kcal- 445, Proteins- 108g, Fats- 1g, Carbs- 1g

Ingredients

1 & 1/2 cups of buttermilk
4 & 1/2 pounds of chicken breast
4 garlic cloves, halved

1/2 teaspoon salt
4 fresh thyme sprigs

How to make Grilled Buttermilk Chicken

Add buttermilk, thyme, garlic, and salt in a large bowl. Add chicken and flip to coat. Store in the refrigerator for 8 hours or overnight. Drain chicken, discarding marinade. Grill covered over medium heat until a thermometer reads 165 ° C, 6-8 minutes on each side.

Spicy Edamame

Servings-1, Kcal- 130, Proteins- 15g, Fats- 2g, Carbs- 12g

Ingredients

16 ounces frozen edamame pods
2 teaspoons of kosher salt
1/4 teaspoon red pepper flakes

1/2 teaspoon garlic powder
3/4 teaspoon ground ginger

How to make Spicy Edamame

Place the Edamame in a large saucepan and cover with water. Bring to a boil. Cover and cook until tender, 4-5 minutes; drain. Put in a large bowl. Add spices; mix to coat.

Cauliflower Mash

Servings-1, Kcal- 70, Proteins- 3g, Fats- 1g, Carbs- 10g

Ingredients

1 large head cauliflower, chopped
1 teaspoon whole peppercorns
1/2 cup chicken broth

1/2 teaspoon salt
2 garlic cloves, crushed
1 bay leaf

How to make Cauliflower Mash

Place the cauliflower in a large saucepan. Add water to cover. Bring to a boil. Lower the temperature and simmer for 10-12 minutes. Drain; return to the pan. In the meantime, mix the remaining ingredients in a small saucepan. Bring to a boil. Remove from the stove immediately and filter; throw away the garlic, peppercorns, and bay leaf. Add the cauliflower broth. Crush to achieve the desired consistency.

Pistachio Salmon

Servings-2, Kcal- 515, Proteins- 80g, Fats- 17g, Carbs- 4g

Ingredients

1/3 cup pistachios, finely chopped
2 tablespoons of panko bread crumb
1/4 cup grated Parmesan cheese

1 salmon fillet (1 pound)
1/2 teaspoon salt
1/4 teaspoon pepper

How to make Pistachio Salmon

Preheat the oven to 200 ° C. Combine the pistachios with breadcrumbs and cheese in a flat bowl. Place salmon on 15 x 10 x 1 inch greased aluminum foil. Skin side down; sprinkle with salt and pepper. Garnish with the pistachio mixture.

Bake uncovered until the fish peels off easily with a fork, 15 to 20 minutes.

Cod and Asparagus Bake

Servings-4, Kcal- 312, Proteins- 60g, Fats- 9g, Carbs- 3g

Ingredients

4 cod fillets (4 ounces each)
1&1/2 teaspoons of grated lemon zest
1/4 cup grated Romano cheese

2 tablespoons of lemon juice
1 pound asparagus, trimmed

How to make Cod and Asparagus Bake

Preheat the oven to 170 C. Add cod and asparagus to a baking pan. Brush the baking pan with oil. Brush the fish with lemon juice. Sprinkle with lemon zest. Sprinkle fish and vegetables with Romano cheese.

Cook for about 12 minutes until the fish peels off easily with a fork. Take the pan out of the oven. Preheat broiler. Broil cod mixture 3-4 inches from the heat until the vegetables are lightly browned, 2-3 minutes.

Sauted Garlic Mushrooms

Servings-2, Kcal- 316, Proteins- 2g, Fats- 34g, Carbs- 5g

Ingredients

3/4 pound sliced fresh mushrooms
2 to 3 teaspoons minced garlic

1 tablespoon bread crumbs
1/3 cup olive oil

How to make Sauted Garlic Mushrooms

Fry mushrooms, garlic, and breadcrumbs in oil in a large pan until the mushrooms are tender

Sauted Radishes with Green Beans

Servings-12, Kcal- 240, Proteins- 3g, Fats- 21g, Carbs- .3g

Ingredients

1 tablespoon olive oil
1/2 pound fresh green beans, trimmed
1 cup thinly sliced radishes

1/2 teaspoon sugar
1/4 teaspoon salt
2 tablespoons of pine nuts

How to make Sauted Radishes with Green Beans

Heat the oil in a large pan over medium to high heat. Add beans; cook and stir for 3-4 minutes or until tender and crispy. Add radishes; Cook for 2 to 3 minutes longer and stir occasionally until the vegetables are tender. Stir in sugar and salt; sprinkle with walnuts.

Green omega 3 boost smoothie

Servings-1, Kcal- 770, Proteins- 25g, Fats- 58g, Carbs- 2g

Ingredients

4 tablespoons of vanilla protein powder
1 Tablespoon flax seeds
2 tablespoons of flaxseed oil
2 tablespoons of MCT oil

Water
4 cups of fresh spinach
1 avocado

How to make Green omega 3 boost smoothie
In a blender, mix all the ingredients. Blend well until smooth. Your smoothie is ready.

Oven-Roasted Salmon

Servings-4, Kcal- 340, Proteins- 70g, Fats- 5g, Carbs- 4g

Ingredients

1 center-cut salmon fillet (1&1/2 pounds)   1/2 teaspoon salt
1 tablespoon olive oil   1/4 teaspoon pepper

How to make Oven-Roasted Salmon

Place a large cast-iron pan or another baking pan in a cold oven. Preheat the oven to 220 C. In the meantime, brush the salmon with oil and sprinkle with salt and pepper.

Carefully remove the pan from the oven. Place the fish face down in a pan. Return to the oven. Cook uncovered until the salmon falls apart slightly and a thermometer shows 125 ° C, 14-18 minutes. Cut the salmon into four equal portions.

Coconut Chai Smoothie

Servings-1, Kcal- 620, Proteins- 24g, Fats- 45g, Carbs- 2g
Ingredients

1cup black tea (chilled)   2 tablespoons of MCT oil
Dash of vanilla extracts   1 cup coconut milk
Pinch of cardamom   4 tablespoons of vanilla protein powder
½ teaspoon cinnamon and ginger (both)

How to make coconut chai smoothie

In a blender, mix all the ingredients. Blend well until smooth. Your smoothie is ready.

Roasted Fresh Okra

Servings-2, Kcal- 200, Proteins- 2g, Fats- 21g, Carbs- 3g

Ingredients

1 pound fresh okra
3 tablespoons of olive oil

1/2 teaspoon salt
1/4 teaspoon pepper

How to make Roasted Fresh Okra

Preheat the oven to 200 °C. Mix the okra with oil, salt, and pepper. Arrange it in a 15x10x1 inch format. Roast for 13 - 17 minutes or until the bottom is tender and slightly golden.

Mediterranean Chicken

Servings-3, Kcal- 650, Proteins- 140g, Fats- 11g, Carbs- 3g

Ingredients

4 boneless chicken breast halves
1/4 teaspoon salt
1/4 teaspoon pepper
16 pitted Greek or ripe olives, sliced

3 tablespoons of olive oil
1 pint grape tomatoes
3 tablespoons of capers

How to make Mediterranean Chicken

Sprinkle chicken with salt and pepper. In a large ovenproof pan, cook the chicken in oil over medium heat until golden brown, 2-3 minutes on each side.

Add tomatoes, olives, and capers. Bake uncovered for 10-14 minutes.

Deviled Chicken

Servings-4, Kcal- 300, Proteins- 50g, Fats- 12g, Carbs- 1g

Ingredients

6 chicken leg quarters
1/4 cup olive oil
1 tablespoon lemon juice
1 teaspoon paprika

1 tablespoon mustard
1 teaspoon salt
1/4 teaspoon pepper

How to make Deviled Chicken

Preheat the oven to 190 °C. Place the chicken in a 15x10x1-in. Pan. Combine other ingredients in a small bowl. Pour over the chicken. Bake uncovered for 50 to 60 minutes.

Lemon-Butter Tilapia with Almonds

Servings-3, Kcal- 380, Proteins- 50g, Fats- 21g, Carbs- 3g

Ingredients

4 tilapia fillets (4 ounces each)
1/2 teaspoon salt
1/4 teaspoon pepper
1/4 cup chicken broth

1 tablespoon olive oil
1/4 cup butter, cubed
2 tablespoons of lemon juice
1/4 cup sliced almonds

How to make Lemon-Butter Tilapia with Almonds

Sprinkle the fillets with salt and pepper. Heat oil over medium heat in a large non-stick pan. Add fillets; cook until the fish peels off easily with a fork, 2-3 minutes on each side. Remove and keep warm.

Add butter, wine, and lemon juice to the same pan; cook and stir until the butter has melted. Serve with fish; Sprinkle with almonds.

Buffalo Chicken Meatballs

Servings-4, Kcal- 345, Proteins- 50g, Fats- 13g, Carbs- 5g

Ingredients

3/4 cup almond flour
1/4 cup chopped celery
1/3 cup plus 1/2 cup Louisiana-style hot sauce
1 pound lean ground chicken

1 large egg white
Reduced-fat blue cheese

How to make Buffalo Chicken Meatballs

Preheat the oven to 200 °C. Mix the flour, 1/3 cup hot sauce, celery, and egg whites in a large bowl. Add chicken; mix lightly but carefully. Form twenty-four 1 inch Balls. Place on a greased rack in a pan. Bake for 20-25 minutes or until cooked. Mix the meatballs with the rest of the hot sauce. If desired, drizzle with dressing just before serving.

Lemon Basil Salmon

Servings-2, Kcal- 200, Proteins- 39g, Fats- 5g, Carbs- 2g

Ingredients

2 salmon fillets (5 ounces each)
1 tablespoon olive oil
1 tablespoon minced fresh basil
Lemon wedges, optional

1 tablespoon lemon juice
1/8 teaspoon pepper
1/8 teaspoon salt

How to make Lemon Basil Salmon

Place each fillet with the skin facing down on an aluminum foil. Combine oil, basil, lemon juice, salt, and pepper. Coat on the salmon. Fold the aluminum foil around the fish and close it tightly.

Cook over a campfire or on a covered grill until the fish peels off easily with a fork (10-15 minutes). Open the aluminum foil carefully so that steam can escape. Serve with lemon wedges if desired.

Lemon-Roasted Asparagus

Servings-2, Kcal- 240, Proteins- 3g, Fats- 23g, Carbs- 5g

Ingredients

2 pounds of fresh asparagus, trimmed
1/4 cup olive oil
4 teaspoons of grated lemon zest

2 garlic cloves, minced
1/2 teaspoon salt
1/2 teaspoon pepper

How to make Lemon-Roasted Asparagus

Preheat the oven to 205 °C. Place asparagus in a greased 15x10x1-inch. pan. Mix the remaining ingredients; Mix to coat. Roast for 8-12 minutes until crispy.

Cinnamon Smoothie

Servings-1, Kcal- 250, Proteins- 3g, Fats- 26g, Carbs- 3g

Ingredients

1/2 cup coconut milk
1/2 cup water + some ice cubes
1 tablespoon MCT oil

1/2 teaspoon cinnamon
1 tablespoon chia seeds
1 teaspoon vanilla extract

How to make Keto Cinnamon Smoothie

Put all the ingredients into a blender. Blend well until smooth. Your smoothie is ready.

Roasted Rosemary Cauliflower

Servings-1, Kcal- 250, Proteins- 3g, Fats- 25g, Carbs- 5g

Ingredients

1 medium head cauliflower florets

2 tablespoons of olive oil

2 teaspoons of rosemary

1/2 teaspoon salt

How to make Roasted Rosemary Cauliflower

Preheat the oven to 200 C. Mix all the ingredients; spread in a greased 15x10x1 inch pan. Roast gently until lightly browned for 20-25 minutes, stirring occasionally.

Marinated Grilled Chicken

Servings-3, Kcal- 400, Proteins- 75g, Fats- 12g, Carbs- 3g

Ingredients

1/4 cup balsamic vinegar

2 tablespoons of olive oil

1-1/2 teaspoons lemon juice

1/2 teaspoon lemon-pepper seasoning

4 boneless skinless chicken breast halves (6 ounces each)

How to make Marinated Grilled Chicken

Combine vinegar, oil, lemon juice, and lemon pepper in a large plastic bag, add chicken. Close the bag. Store in the refrigerator for 30 minutes.

Drain and throw away the marinade. Moisten a paper towel with cooking oil; using long-handled tongs, lightly coat the grill rack. Grill over medium heat for 5-7 minutes per side or until the thermometer shows 170 °.

Pressure electric cooker pot bourbon chicken

Servings-4, Kcal- 362, Proteins- 85g, Fats- 1g, Carbs- 4g

Ingredients

1 chopped garlic clove
1 teaspoon ground ginger
1 teaspoon paprika flakes
2 tablespoons of ketchup
2 tablespoons of cornstarch

1/4 cup apple juice
1 tablespoon apple cider vinegar
1/2 cup water
1/3 cup soy sauce
2 tablespoons of cold water

2 lb boneless Skinless chicken breast cut into 1 - 2 inch pieces

How to make Pressure electric cooker pot bourbon chicken

In an instant pot, add your chicken, garlic, ginger, red pepper flakes, apple juice, tomato sauce, vinegar, water, and soy sauce. Stir to combine. Put the lid on the instant container and close it. Set in the manual configuration for 5 minutes. Remove the chicken from the instant pot. Turn your instant pot into sauté mode. In a small bowl, combine the cornstarch and cold water and beat the sauce on the bottom of the bowl until it is thick. Stir chicken well. Serve

Baked vegetables

Servings-2, Kcal- 100, Proteins- 0g, Fats- 12g, Carbs- 7g

Ingredients

1 tablespoon / 30 ml cooking oil   Salt and pepper
1 pound / 0.5 kg vegetables (broccoli, cauliflower, parsnips, zucchini, etc.), evenly chopped

How to make Baked vegetables

Preheat oven for about 5 minutes at 182 ° C. Chop vegetables, mix with oil, salt and pepper. Place the vegetables in the oven and bake for 15 - 20 minutes, stirring the vegetables every 5 - 8 minutes. Some vegetables need more time and others need less - use your judgment when opening the tray to stir vegetables. You want the exterior to be golden and crisp and the interior to be delicate.

Buffalo cauliflower

Servings-2, Kcal- 115, Proteins- 1g, Fats- 11g, Carbs- 2g

Ingredients

1 cauliflower, cut into 1 1/2 "florets
2-3 tablespoons of nutrient yeast
2-3 tablespoons of Frank red hot sauce
1 1/2 teaspoons of sweetener

1 tablespoon corn starch
2 teaspoons of avocado oil
1/4 teaspoon sea salt

How to make buffalo cauliflower

Preheat the oven to 200 degrees C. Lay out a baking tray with non-stick parchment paper. Add all the ingredients except cauliflower in a bowl. Marinate cauliflower with the mixture. Spread the cauliflower evenly on a baking sheet. Bake for 40 minutes, cook until the cauliflower has golden brown edges.

Spicy kale chips

Servings-2, Kcal- 60, Proteins- 0g, Fats- 6g, Carbs- 1g

Ingredients

3 cups of kale
1 tablespoon olive oil

½ - 1 teaspoon sea salt
1 - 2 tablespoons of Za'atar spice

How to cook spicy kale chips

Put your washed and dried kale in a large bowl and mix with olive oil. Add the spices and mix well. Place the kale in the oven, set at 170 ° C.

The chips should be ready when the edges are brown but not burnt. Be sure to have an eye (and nose) on them while cooking. It should take about 10-15 minutes in a preheated oven.

Air Fried Bagels

8 servings: Calories: 166| Protein: 10 g | Carbs: 27 g | Fat: 2 g
Ingredients:
Whole wheat flour(2 cups)   Plain Greek yogurt (2 cups)
Kosher salt (1 t.)   Eggs, beaten (1)
Baking powder (1 tbsp.)

Directions:

Flour, baking soda, and salt should all be measured out and whisked in a bowl. Mix in the yogurt by stirring with a spoon or rubber spatula. Create a dough ball on a floured surface.Cut the dough into eight portions. To form a bagel shape, roll every piece into an eight to ten-inch rope and squeeze the sides together.

Your preferred bagel toppings should be sprinkled on after brushing with beaten egg. Elevate your air fryer to 350 degrees Fahrenheit (10-12 min.) or until golden to air fry the bagels. Before slicing, let cool for five minutes.

Avocado Tempura

2 servings: Calories: 428| Carbs: 35 g | Protein: 8 g | Fat: 28 g

Ingredients:
Avocados (2)   pepper and salt
Seasoned panko breadcrumbs (0.75 cups)   Olive oil spray

Directions:
Set the fryer temperature to 375° Fahrenheit/191° Celsius to preheat. Remove the avocado's skin and seed by slicing it in half. Push avocado halves into breadcrumbs on a plate until they are thoroughly coated on all sides. If desired, softly sprinkle the skin with virgin avocado oil spray. Air fry the prepared avocados for seven minutes to serve.

Banana Vegan French Toast

2 servings:Calories: 226| Carbs: 39 g |Protein: 5 g |Fat: 5 g

Ingredients:

Sourdough bread (4-5 slices)   Almond milk (1 cup)
Banana, mashed (1)   Cinnamon (1 tbsp.)

Directions:

Warm the fryer unit at 430° Fahrenheit/221° Celsius. The banana should be well mashed in a big bowl so that there are almost no pieces. Then, blend in the cinnamon and milk.Thoroughly coat all sides of the bread with the mixture. Place them inside the air fryer on foil or parchment paper to cook till crispy (7-8 min.).

Anti Inflammatory Spice Smoothie

Servings-2, Kcal- 460, Proteins- 24g, Fats- 30g, Carbs- 3g
Ingredients

Water   1 cup blueberries
4 tablespoons of vanilla protein powder   2 tablespoons of MCT oil
2 tablespoons of flaxseed oil   2 avocados
½ teaspoon cinnamon, ginger, turmeric (each)

Directions:

In a blender, mix all the ingredients. Blend well until smooth. Your smoothie is ready.

Polenta Fries

3 servings: Calories: 80| Carbs: 17 g| Fat: 0 g | Protein: 2 g

Ingredients:

Prepare polenta, 1 pack (16 oz.)   Pepper and salt
Non-stick olive oil cooking spray (as required)

Directions:

Achieve a 350 degrees Fahrenheit air fryer temperature (175 degrees Celsius). French fry-like long, thin polenta slices should be cut out. Cooking spray should be applied to the basket's bottom. Toss half of the fries with pepper and salt into the fryer basket with the tops spritzed with a little cooking spray to air fry (10 min.). With a spatula, turn the fries over. Prepare them further till they are crispy as desired (5 min.). Move fries to a platter covered with a layer of paper towels to absorb any leftover fats. Lastly, proceed with the second batch of fries.

Chicken Tenderloin

6 servings: Calories: 200| Carbs: 4 g | Fat: 7 g |Protein: 30 g

Ingredients:

Chicken tenderloins (1 lb.)   Italian seasoning (1 t.)
Olive oil (2 tbsp.)   Salt (0.5 t.)
Garlic powder (0.5 t.)   Smoked paprika (1 t.)

Directions:

Set the fryer's temperature to 375° Fahrenheit/191° Celsius. Lubricate the fryer basket sparingly.Chicken tenders - as well as oil and seasonings - should be combined in a mixing dish till they are thoroughly blended.

One layer of chicken tenders should be added to the fryer basket with seven to eight minutes of air frying, flipping halfway through the cooking cycle.The tenderloins should be taken from the fryer basket and given five minutes to rest before being served.

Orange Creamsicle Smoothie

Servings-1, Kcal- 720, Proteins- 24g, Fats- 60g, Carbs- 3g
Ingredients

4 tablespoons of vanilla protein powder
2 tablespoons of MCT oil
½ - 1 teaspoon orange zest minced

Water
½ cup heavy cream.
1 avocado

Directions:

In a blender, mix all the ingredients. Blend well until smooth. Your smoothie is ready.

Harissa Veggie Fries

2 portions: Calories:250| Carbs: 45 g | Fat: 6 g | Protein: 3 g

Ingredients:
Sweet potatoes (400 g).   Harissa (2 t.)
Olive oil (2 t.)

Directions:

Preheat the air fryer at 180° Fahrenheit/82 ° Celsius. Thoroughly wash and peel the potatoes, removing the peel if desired. Toss the sweet potato wedges in the harissa and olive oil. Arrange the wedges in the fryer basket to air fry (15 min.) tossing halfway through its cooking cycle to serve.

Crispy Chicken Bites

4 servings: Calories: 268| Carbs: 30 g | Protein: 20 g | Fat: 7 g

Ingredients:

Chicken breasts – (2)   Eggs (2)
Olive oil (1 t.)   Pepper (1 t.)
Italian seasoning (1 t.)   Smoked paprika (0.5 t.)
Breadcrumbs (1 and 0.5 cups)   Whole wheat flour (0.25 cups)

Directions:

Set the fryer's temperature to 390° Fahrenheit/199° Celsius. Whenever necessary, lubricate the fryer basket using non-stick cooking oil. Slice the chicken into edible bites. Whisk the egg. Mash the breadcrumbs, spices, and flour. Mix in the oil with the chicken bites and gently toss. After that, coat each chicken bite thoroughly by dipping it into the egg, followed by the breadcrumb mixture. Put the chicken pieces in the fryer basket – single-layered. Air fry till the meat reaches 165° Fahrenheit/74° Celsius (8-10 min.). Serve the chicken bites with your preferred dipping sauce after carefully removing them from the fryer unit.

Louisiana Style Prawns

5 portions: Calories: 160| Carbs: 2 g | Fat: 8 g | Protein: 20 g
Ingredients:

Cajun seasoning (1 tbsp.)   olive oil (3 tbsp.)
Shrimp: frozen, raw, peeled & deveined (1 lb.).   Garlic

Directions:

Set the air fryer temperature at 400° Fahrenheit/204° Celsius. The bottom of the fryer should be filled with frozen shrimp. Cajun seasoning should be added to the shrimp. Top the shrimp with the oil and garlic. Air fry for five minutes. Stir the shrimp, oil, and spices with a spoon. To finish cooking the shrimp, air fry them for five to six more minutes. Add parsley, Cajun seasoning sprinklings, or lemon wedges as garnishes.

Crunchy Ranch Chicken

4 portions: Calories: 400 | Carbs: 5 g | Protein: 70g | Fat: 10g

Ingredients:

Chicken wings (2 lb.)   Baking powder (1 tbsp.)
Ranch seasoning mix (2 tbsp. from 1 pkg.)

Directions:

If the chicken wings are not already divided, make wings and
drumettes out of them. Throw away the wing tips. Dab the chicken dry
with a wad of disposable/paper towels. Put the wings in a zipped bag
or a big bowl. Gently toss the wings to combine after adding the
baking powder and ranch seasoning blend. Add the wings to the fryer
in a single layer. After 10 minutes of air frying at 360°
Fahrenheit/182° Celsius, turn the food over. Then, raise the
temperature to 400° Fahrenheit/204° Celsius and fry for an additional
six minutes. To ensure the wings are heated to a temperature of 165°
Fahrenheit/74° Celsius, use an instant-read thermometer.

Jamaican Chicken Fajitas

4 portions: Calories: 186| Carbs: 6 g | Fat: 7 g | Protein: 25 g

Ingredients:

Olive oil (1 tbsp.)   Pepper and salt (as desired)
Sliced chicken breasts (2)   Lime (1)
Taco seasoning (1 t.)   Sliced red onion (0.25 cup)

Directions:

Set the fryer to 390° Fahrenheit/199° Celsius before using. Sliced
items should be combined with seasonings and oil in a mixing
container. Add them to the fryer basket. Air fry till the chicken reaches
165° Fahrenheit or 74° Celsius – internal temperature (15 min.). Serve
after adding cilantro and lime juice.

Turkey & Mushroom Sandwich

5 portions: Calories: 191| Carbs: 4 g | Fat: 9 g | Protein: 23 g

Ingredients:

Lean ground turkey (1 lb.)
Fresh mushrooms, medium (8)
Cilantro, chopped (0.25 cup)
Worcestershire sauce (1 tbsp.)

Olive oil spray (as needed)
Kosher salt (0.5 t.)
Black pepper (0.25 t.)
Onion & garlic powder (1 t. each)

Directions:

Before placing the mushrooms in your food processor, thoroughly rinse them with water and shake off any excess water. Puree. Place the shredded turkey, cilantro, and each of the seasonings in a big mixing container along with the pureed mushrooms.

Mix thoroughly with your hands. Five patties are created by dividing the turkey burger mixture. To keep the burgers from compacting themselves in the middle, make an indentation with your thumb in the middle of each one. The turkey patties should be sprayed with frying oil spray on both sides.

Chinese Garlic Prawns

Servings-1, Kcal- 20, Proteins- 0g, Fats- 0.5g, Carbs- 4 g

Ingredients

2 cups of boiled water
1 tea bag
1 strawberry
1 slice of lemon

1 stevia
1 tablespoon apple cider vinegar
ice cubes

How to make Berry lemonade

Boil water in a pan. Brew your tea in mugs with the boiled water. Cut a strawberry into small pieces and add it in your tea with a slice of lemon. Add ice cubes and stevia. Mix properly.

Creole Trout

6 servings: Calories: 168| Carbs: 2 g | Protein: 24 g |Fat: 7 g

Ingredients:
Steelhead trout fillets (1.5 lb.)   Fresh lime or lemon
Seafood rub (1 tbsp.)

Directions:

Put some seafood rub on the trout's top. Unless the fish has no skin, leave the skin on. Once the fish is done, it will be simple to remove. If your fryer needs to be warmed up, set it to 400 degrees Fahrenheit.

Arrange the trout in the fryer tray with the skin-side facing downward. Oil can be brushed on or sprayed on if you choose, but it is not required. The trout should be thoroughly done after 8 to 10 minutes of air frying. Serve the fish right away with your chosen sides and a drizzle of fresh lime or lemon juice.

Fiery Prawns

3 servings: Calories: 194| Protein: 25 g | Carbs - 3.1 g | Fat: 9 g

Ingredients:
Shrimp – raw - jumbo (1 lb.)   Garlic powder (0.5 t.)
Olive oil (2 tbsp.)   Tabasco sauce (1 t.)
Water (2 tbsp.)   Dried parsley (0.5 t.)
Red pepper flakes (1 t.)   Onion salt (0.5 t.)
Smoked paprika (0.5 t.)   Oregano - dried (1 t.)
Black pepper (0.5 t.)

Directions:

Discard the veins and shells from the shrimp. Toss all the fixings – except the shrimp - into a resealable plastic bag to combine.
Add the shrimp and fully shake till coated. Pop them into the fridge to marinate (4-6 hr.). Then add to the fryer unit to cook till they are pink (10 min.). Serve with your favorite side.

Lemon-Pepper Haddock

2 servings: Calories: 250| Protein: 50 g | Carbs: 1 g | Fat: 4g

Ingredients:
Haddock (1 lb.)
Onion powder (0.5 t.)
Paprika (0.5 t. to 1 t.)

Cayenne pepper (0.25 t.)
Garlic powder (1 t.)

Directions:

To blend the fish seasoning, combine the seasoning; then, set aside. Dry off the haddock fillets using paper towels. Brush the haddock with oil, sprinkle it with seasoning, flip it over, and continue.

Place the fillets in the fryer gently. For 8-10 minutes, air fry them at 350°Fahrenheit/180°Celsius. The fillets do not need to be turned over.

Pistachio-Crusted Salmon Fillet

2 serving: Calories: 565| Protein: 65 g | Carbs: 5 g | Fat:25

Ingredients:

Pistachios, finely chopped (0.25 cup)
Salmon fillet (1 lb.)

Mustard (1-2 tbsp.)
Garlic powder (1 t.)

Directions:

Take the salmon from the box and use paper towels to pat it dry. Rub the salmon with the mustard using a spoon or brush. Add some garlic powder. Pistachios should be finely chopped and uniformly distributed over the salmon.

As you prepare the salmon, warm your fryer to 390° Fahrenheit and allow it to run for five minutes if it does not have a preheat option. Spray some non-stick spray on your basket. Salmon should be inserted skin-side down. Depending on how you prefer your salmon cooked, air fry it for anywhere between 9 to 12 minutes.

Rosemary Catfish

2 serving: Calories: 570| Protein: 55 g | Carbs: 28 g | Fat: 4 g

Ingredients:

Catfish fillet (1 lb.)

Rosemary (1 tbsp.)

Fish fry seasoning (1 cup)

Cooking spray (1 tbsp.)

Directions:

Set the fryer to 400° Fahrenheit/204° Celsius to warm up (5 min.). While waiting, skin, clean, and filet the catfish. Use paper towels to pat the fillets dry. Dredge the dried fillets in the spices after adding the fish fry spice to a shallow dish. For a light, equal coating on both sides, gently press the fillets into the seasonings. Put the breaded fish in the fryer basket that has been preheated. Now, add a thin layer of cooking spray to the top of each piece. After that, air fry for 20 minutes in the heated unit. With a spatula, gently flip the fillets over after 10 minutes, lightly coat the other side, and continue to air fry (10 min.). Serve warm.

Instant Pot Chicken Soup

Servings-6, Kcal- 275, Proteins- 57g, Fats- 4g, Carbs- 3g

Ingredients

1 whole chicken

2 tablespoons Italian spice

5 chopped celery stalks

2 liters of water

2 medium carrots, chopped

2 tablespoons of salt

1 medium onion, chopped

1 teaspoon black pepper

3 garlic cloves, peeled and chopped

1/4 cup parsley chopped

How to make instant pot chicken soup

Place every ingredient (except parsley) in an instant pot. Put Instant Pot on manual high pressure for 25 minutes. Release the pressure slowly and enjoy it. Garnish with parsley.

Chocolate Cauliflower Smoothie

Servings-1, Kcal- 308, Proteins- 15g, Fats- 23g, Carbs- 14g

Ingredients

1 cup of unsweetened almond milk	1 tablespoon of cacao nibs
1 cup of frozen cauliflower florets	3 tablespoons of hemp seeds
1.5 tablespoons of cocoa powder	pinch of sea salt

How to make Chocolate cauliflower breakfast smoothie

Combine all the ingredients in a blender and blend until smooth.

Cinnamon Roasted Pumpkin

2 portions: Calories: 160| Carbs: 22 g | Fat: 7 g | Protein: 3 g

Ingredients:

Avocado or olive oil (1 tbsp.)	Kosher salt (0.5 t.)
Ground cinnamon (0.5 t.)	Garlic powder (0.25 t.)
Sugar pumpkin or another variety (2 lb.)	

Directions:

Set the heating temperature of the fryer at 380° Fahrenheit/194° Celsius. Peel and cube the pumpkin into ¾-inch pieces. Scoop the pumpkin into a bowl and mix in the seasonings and oil. Add the seasoned pumpkin to the fryer and scatter in a single layer or prepare in batches if needed (18-20 min.). Shake the basket at about 10 minutes into the air fryer.

Mushroom & Broccoli Casserole Favorite

4 servings: Calories: 72| Protein: 2 g | Carbs: 8 g | Fat: 3 g

Ingredients:

Broccoli florets (6 oz./about 3 cups)

Whole mushrooms (8 oz./about 3 cups)

Pearl onions (6 oz./about 1.25 cups)

Olive oil (2 t.)

Salt (as desired)

Garlic (2 t.)

Thyme (1 t.)

Directions:

Preheat the air fryer to reach 400° Fahrenheit or 204° Celsius. Rinse and dab dry each of the veggies. Slice any larger sized mushrooms into quarters or smaller ones into halves for equal air frying. Toss them in the basket and add broccoli and onions. Drizzle and lightly toss oil over the vegetables.

Mince and add garlic, thyme, and salt. Spray the air fryer basket with a small portion of cooking oil/spray and add the prepared vegetables to cook (3 min.). Now, stir, and cook until they are fork-tender (+ 3 min.).

Mustard Honey Thighs

4 servings: Calories: 410| Protein: 19 g | Carbs: 2 g | Fat: 27 g

Ingredients:

Chicken thighs (1 lb.)

Honey (0.33 or 1/3 cup)

Olive oil (2 tbsp.)

Cooking spray/oil

Dijon mustard (0.33 cup)

Directions:

Warm the fryer at 400° Fahrenheit or 204° Celsius. Lightly spritz the basket with the spray. Prepare the sauce components and rub it thoroughly over the chicken pieces. Arrange them in the basket with the skin-side upward to air fry till its internal temperature reaches 165° Fahrenheit or 74° Celsius (14 min.). Enjoy as a meal or snack for up to five days.

Chicken Tandoori Tikka Masala

2 portions: Calories: 234 | Carbs: 7 g | Fat: 4 g | Protein: 40 g

Ingredients:

Chicken breasts (10 oz.)
Onion (1 red)
Tandoori masala (1 tbsp.)
Ginger & ginger (1 tbsp. each)
Red chilli powder (1 t.)

olive oil cooking spray
Greek yogurt (0.5 cup)
Garlic (1 tbsp.)
Kashmiri red pepper (2 t.)

Directions:

First, mince the garlic and ginger. Whisk the marinade ingredients in a mixing container (spices, garlic, ginger, and yogurt). Next cube (removing all fat & bones) and toss in the chicken to the marinade - tossing fulling. Now, add onions to marinate (20-30 min.). Preheat the air fryer at 390° Fahrenheit/199° Celsius. Lastly arrange the chicken to the fryer basket - single layered. Lightly mist it with cooking oil spray and air fry (20 min.). Flip it over at the ten-minute marker. Serve the chicken with some freshly squeezed lemon juice or as desired.

Prosciutto-Wrapped Chicken Breast

4 portions: Calories: 260| Carbs: 1- g | Protein: 44 g | Fat: 8 g

Ingredients:

Chicken breasts (3 whole)
Pepper & salt (to taste)

Sage (2 t.)
Prosciutto (8 oz.)

Directions:

Warm the air fryer at 400° Fahrenheit/204° Celsius. Remove all the bones from the chicken breasts and place them onto a chopping block. Dust it with sage, salt (approx. 1/4 t.), and pepper. Wrap each breast with prosciutto (2-3 slices) to enclose most of the chicken. Cook for 15 minutes, turning once. The temperature of the chicken should reach 160° Fahrenheit/71° Celsius or above. If not, return it to the air fryer for another two to six minutes. When done, wait about five minutes to serve.

Thyme & Rosemary Fried Chicken Legs

4 servings: Calories: 440| Protein: 26 g | Net Carbs: 1 g | Fat: 30 g

Ingredients:

Olive oil (0.25 cup)   Fresh thyme (1 t.) or dried (0.25 t.)
Garlic (3 cloves)   Fresh rosemary (2 t.) or dried (0.5 t.)
Chicken legs (4. 1.5 lb.)   Lemon: Zested (1 t.) + Juice (1 tbsp.)
Salt & pepper (.125 or 1/8 t. each)

Directions:
Preheat the air fryer to 400° Fahrenheit/204° Celsius. Mince the garlic and thyme or rosemary. Zest and juice the lemon. Combine oil with the rosemary, garlic, thyme, lemon juice, and zest. Then, spread one teaspoon of the butter mixture under the skin of each chicken thigh.

Spread remaining butter over the skin of each thigh and dust with pepper and salt. Place the prepared chicken, skin side upward, on a lightly greased tray in the fryer basket to air fry (20 min.), turning once. Turn chicken again (skin side up) and cook until a thermometer reads 170° Fahrenheit/77° Celsius to 175° Fahrenheit/79 ° Celsius (5 min.) to serve.

Air Fried Mussels

4 servings: Calories: 223| Protein: 27 g | Carbs: 8 g | Fat: 8 g

Ingredients:

Mussels (1 lb.)   olive oil (1 tbsp.)
Water (1 cup)   Garlic (2 t.)
Parsley, basil & chives (1 t. each)

Directions:
Warm the air fryer to 390° Fahrenheit/199° Celsius. Clean your mussels by soaking for ½ hour. Brush and clean them to eliminate the outer layer which covers the mussels. Mince the garlic. Combine the water, butter, garlic, chives, basil, parsley, and mussels in the pan and place in the fryer unit. Set the time for three minutes, check, and see if the mussels are opened. If they are not opened, continue to air fry an additional two minutes.

Breaded Scallops

2 servings: Calories: 375| Protein: 42 g | Carbs: 15 g | Fat: 16g

Ingredients:
crackers/Ritz (0.5 cup)

Seafood seasoning - Old Bay (0.5 t.)

Sea scallops (1 lb.)

Garlic powder (0.5 t.)

Olive oil (2 tbsp.)

Cooking spray

Directions:
Preheat the air fryer to 390° Fahrenheit/199° Celsius. Finely crush and combine the crackers with garlic powder and seafood seasoning. Add the oil in a second shallow bowl. Dab dry and dip each scallop in oil, then dredge it through the breading till it is thoroughly coated.

Set aside and continue with the remaining scallops. Lightly spritz the fryer basket with cooking spray. Lastly arrange scallops in the prepared basket, so that they are not touching; working in batches if needed. Now air fry for two minutes. Gently flip the scallops with a small spatula and cook until opaque .

Crab Legs

1 serving: Calories: 320| Protein: 22 g | Carbs: -0- g | Fat: 23 g

Ingredients:
Snow crab legs (1 cluster)

Cajun seasoning (1 tbsp.)

Olive oil (2 tbsp.)

Optional:
Lemon wedges

Old Bay Seasoning

Melted butter

Directions:
Preheat the fryer unit at 350° Fahrenheit/177° Celsius. Toss the crab legs with olive oil and seasoning. Transfer them into the air fryer to cook (3-5 min.) and serve.

Cajun Jumbo Shrimp

4 servings: Calories: 131| Protein: 22 g | Carbs: 2 g | Fat: 3 g

Ingredients:

Shrimp - cleaned (1 lb.)   Olive oil (1 tbsp.)
Cajun seasoning (2 tbsp.)   Black pepper (0.25 t.)
Kosher salt (0.5 t.)

Remainder of spices @ 1 t. each:

Dried thyme, Garlic powder, Paprika,Cayenne pepper or Chili powder, Onion powder

Directions:

Peel away the outer shell and remove shrimp tails. Then, gently slice the back of the shrimp to remove its black vein. Rinse and place the shrimp on a layer of disposable towels to remove any excess moisture. Warm the air fryer unit at 370° Fahrenheit/188 ° Celsius.

Add shrimp to a big mixing container and toss with oil and seasonings till they are evenly coated. Place the prepared shrimp in the fryer basket, not stacking, to air fry for eight minutes. Shake the basket halfway through for even cooking. Serve immediately while they are hot.

Vegetarian Pizza

1 serving: Calories: 360| Protein: 12 g | Carbs: 35- g | Fat: 18 g

Ingredients:

Pita or naan bread (1)   Pizza sauce (3 tbsp.)
Shredded mozzarella cheese (0.5 cup)   Olives (2 tbsp.)

Directions:

Thaw the dough in the oven for 2-3 minutes at 350° Fahrenheit/177° Celsius. Top the pita with pizza sauce and add the cheese. Slice the olives in half and add to the pizza. Put the pizza into the fryer basket. Bake until the cheese is melted (3 min.). Wait for one to two minutes, top with basil, and serve to enjoy.

Calamari Rings

4 servings: Calories: 338 | Carbs: 47 g | Protein: 22 g | Fat: 5 g

Ingredients:
Calamari (300 g/10.6 oz.)
Pita bread (1)
Lemon juice (1 tbsp.)
Dill (0.5 t.)
Eggs (3 - beaten)
whole wheat flour (200 g/7.05 0z.)
Parsley (1 tbsp.)
Pepper & salt (to your liking)
Optional: Baking spray – olive oil used (as required)

Directions:

Warm the fryer unit at 360° Fahrenheit/182° Celsius. Whisk the eggs in a mixing container with the lemon juice. Measure and add flour into another bowl with pepper and salt. Break the pita apart and feed into the blender. Once prepared, add the breadcrumbs in a bowl with salt, pepper, parsley, and dill. Dry the thawed calamari rings using a kitchen towel. Load the rings into the egg bowl, then flour, and lastly the breadcrumbs making sure each layer is well coated. Load the rings into the fryer basket - single layered - to air fry (8 min.). Flip and respray with oil - cook for the same time and temp - to serve.

Air Fryer Parsnips

4 portions: Calories: 94 | Carbs: 17 g | Fat: 2 g | Protein: 2 g

Ingredients:
Parsnips (1 lb.)
Paprika - Garlic and onion powder (0.5 t. each)
Olive oil (1 t.)
Salt (1 t.)

Directions:

Heat the fryer at 390° Fahrenheit/199° Celsius. Wash your parsnips and peel - as you would a carrot – discarding the top and ends. Next cut the parsnips into strips, tossing them into a mixing bowl with a spritz of oil. Sprinkle the seasonings over the parsnips while dusting to cover. Arrange them in the fryer basket (not overlapping). Air fry them until tender and golden to serve (10 min.).

Parsley & Garlic Fried Shrimp

2 servings: Calories: 135| Protein: 28g | Carbs: 2 g | Fat: 2 g

Ingredients:

Jumbo shrimp (20 frozen)
Garlic powder (0.5 t.)
Paprika (0.5 t.)
Flat leaf parsley (1 tbsp.)

Olive oil (1 t.)
Salt (0.25 t.)
Pepper (0.125 or 1/8 t.)

Directions:

Preheat the air fryer at 400° Fahrenheit/204° Celsius (5 min.). Finely chop the parsley. Cook and peel the shrimp. Then, toss all the spice fixings and add the shrimp (in an oversized plastic bag). Pour in oil. Securely close the bag and massage the shrimp to spread the seasoning evenly. Place on a plate at room temperature (1 hr.). Add the shrimp to the basket to cook (2 min.). Next, gently shake the shrimp a bit, and return to the fryer to continue cooking (2 min.). At that time, if not fully heated, continue at one-minute intervals in the fryer till ready. When the shrimps are done, serve it with a sprinkle of parsley to serve.

Grilled Apple & Brie Sandwich

2 sandwiches: Calories: 281 |Carbs: 40 g | Protein: 10 g | Fat: 9

Ingredients:

Multigrain bread (4 slices)
Brie (2 oz.)
Olive oil or spray (as required)

Honey mustard (2 t.)
Crispy apple (half of 1 small)

Directions:

Heat the air fryer at 350° Fahrenheit or 177° Celsius (10 min.). Lightly spritz the basket with cooking spray. Slice the chilled brie and thinly slice the apple. Lay the sliced bread on a platter to spread the mustard on two slices. Portion the fixings between the two sandwiches and layer on top of the mustard, and then top with the other slices of bread. Thoroughly spritz/coat the outer sides of the bread with oil. Transfer to the prepared basket (6 min.). Flip them over and continue cooking until the tops are evenly browned (2 min.). Let them slightly cool (1-2 min.) before slicing and serving.

Lentil Tacos

6 tacos: Calories: 280| Protein: 12 g | Carbs: 28 g | Fat: 13 g

Ingredients:
Hard taco shells (6)
Fajita or taco seasoning (2 t.)
Shredded iceberg lettuce (handful).
Sour cream (2 tbsp.)

Lentils (15 oz. can/400g)
Grated cheese (0.25 cup/25 g)
Tomato (1 medium)
Chives (1 tbsp.)

Directions:
Preheat the air fryer at 360° Fahrenheit/182° Celsius. Drain and thoroughly rinse the lentils. Prepare the lentil filling. Add the lentils to a big mixing container with the taco seasoning - tossing till it's fully coated. Arrange the taco shells in the fryer basket.

Scoop in the mixture (2 tbsp. - heaping for each taco). Top it off with cheese. Air fry till the shells are super crunchy and cheese is gooey (5 min.). Shred the lettuce and discard the seeds to finely chop the tomato. Top the taco off with lettuce, tomato, sour cream, and chives to serve.

Chili Edamame

4 portions: Calories: 110| Protein: 8 g | Carbs: 14 g | Fat: 2g

Ingredients:
Oil (1 tbsp.)
Frozen edamame - in shell (10 oz.)
Sea salt (as desired)

Garlic powder (0.5 t.)
Chili flakes (0.25 tsp.)

Directions:
Warm the air fryer at 390° Fahrenheit or 199° Celsius. Toss the frozen edamame, oil, salt, garlic powder, and red chili flakes in a mixing container. Scatter it into the fryer basket to cook (10 min.). Shake the basket after 5-6 minutes. Then, continue to air fry for the remaining time. Scoop it into a serving bowl with a sprinkle of chili flakes if you desire.

Carrot Crisps

Serving:4: Calories: 125| Carbs: 20 g | Protein: -2- g | Fat: 4 g

Ingredients:
Olive oil (3 tbsp.)   Raw carrot chips (16 oz. pkg.)
Dry ranch dressing mix (1 tbsp.)

Directions:

Program the air fryer at 400° Fahrenheit/204° Celsius. Slice and prepare the carrot chips with oil in a resealable bag. Shake well till covered and dust with the ranch seasoning. Air-fry until crispy (10-12 min.). *Note*: Pause every three minutes to give the air fryer basket a shake.

Chive-Roasted sweet Potatoes

4 portions: Calories: 290| Carbs: 62 g | Fat: 4 g | Protein: 3 g

Ingredients:
sweet potatoes (2 lb.)   Cooking oil spray
Pepper and salt   olive oil (5 tbsp.)
Fresh chives (2 tbsp.)

Directions:

Preheat the air fryer at 400° Fahrenheit/204° Celsius. Lightly spritz the fryer basket with cooking spray. Equally slice the potatoes for best results. Toss them with the oil, pepper, and salt. Scoop them into the fryer to cook (10 min.) flipping halfway through the time.

Finely chop the chives. At that time, check for tenderness, then air fry till the potatoes are fork tender (3-5 min.). Scoop them into an oversized container to toss with chives. Serve them piping hot.

ONE LAST THING

If you enjoyed this book or found it helpful. Please help us by writing a short review on Amazon. Your support makes a difference, and I read your reviews personally. So I can get your feedback and make this book even better.

To leave a review, go to Amazon and type **Anti-Inflammatory Guide and Cookbook for Beginners**. Click on the book to find the review option at the bottom of the page.

Thanks a lot for your support.

About Author

Vania Higgins is a dedicated health and wellness expert with a passion for educating others on the benefits of anti-inflammatory living. Her experience as a certified nutritionist has given her a deep understanding of the impact that food and lifestyle choices have on overall health. In her book, Vania shares her expertise on the topic of inflammation and its impact on our health. With a focus on evidence-based research and practical solutions, she offers readers a comprehensive guide to reducing inflammation and promoting optimal health.

But Vania's passion for anti-inflammatory living goes beyond just the physical benefits. She understands the profound impact that chronic inflammation can have on mental health and overall well-being. With this in mind, she offers readers a comprehensive guide to reducing inflammation in all areas of life. With her guidance, readers will be equipped to make sustainable, life-changing improvements to their health and well-being.

Printed in Great Britain
by Amazon

22545470R00081